The
American Yoga Association
Wellness Book

Also by Alice Christensen:

The American Yoga Association Beginner's Manual

20-Minute Yoga Workouts

Easy Does It Yoga for Older People

The Easy Does It Yoga Trainer's Guide

Meditation

Reflections of Love

The Light of Yoga

The Joy of Celibacy

Conversations with Swami Lakshmanjoo, Volume I
Aspects of Kashmir Shaivism

Conversations with Swami Lakshmanjoo, Volume II
The Yamas and Niyamas of Patanjali

Basic Yoga (videotape)

Complete Relaxation and Meditation (audiotape)

Conversations with Swami Lakshmanjoo (three-videotape set)

The "I Love You" Meditation Technique (audio- and videotape)

The
American Yoga
Association
Wellness Book

Alice Christensen • Founder, American Yoga Association

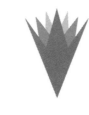

AMERICAN
Y·O·G·A
ASSOCIATION

KENSINGTON BOOKS

Important Note to Readers

The suggestions and techniques in this book are not meant to constitute or substitute for professional medical advice. You should consult your physician before attempting any new fitness program. The author, the American Yoga Association, and the publisher assume no responsibility for injuries suffered while practicing these techniques. The techniques in this book are not recommended for pregnant or nursing women or children under 16. If you experience any discomfort while practicing these techniques, consult your physician.

The models in this book are students of the American Yoga Association.

Photographs by Herbert Ascherman, Jr.

ISBN 1-57566-025-3

KENSINGTON BOOKS are published by

Kensington Publishing Corp.
850 Third Avenue
New York, NY 10022

Design by Carol Tornatore
Composition by Hunter Chisholm,
Protean Solutions

Printed in the United States of America
First Edition: April 1996

10 9 8 7 6 5 4 3 2 1

Acknowledgments

Many people have helped to make this book possible. I would especially like to thank Linda Gajevski for developing and managing the project; Pattie Cerar for her long hours of research; Patricia Rockwood and Anne Wardwell for excellent help with writing and editing; Cynthia Ingalls for sharp-eyed proofreading; Dr. Scott Gerson for kindly reviewing the manuscript from a medical perspective; and the Yoga students who participated in the photography for this book or provided valuable administrative support: Brenda Brown, Kirste Carlson, Sherry Dilley, Corrine Goodman, Carol Goodwin, Carole Guerin, Sue Kraus, David McDowell, Chuck Rosenman, Dan Tickten, Joy Walworth, and Ed Wardwell.

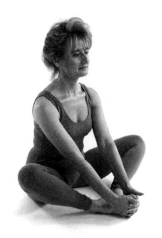

Chapter 14: Pain Management   126

Chapter 15: Premenstrual Syndrome and Menopause   134

Chapter 16: Weight Management   145

Dedication

To Swami Rama of Haridwar and Swami Lakshmanjoo of Kashmir — two great Yoga masters whose strength, health, energy, and wisdom continue to inspire and support me in my life and work in Yoga.

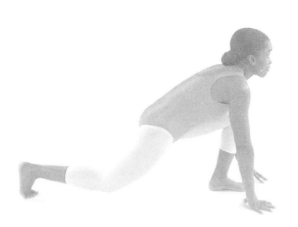

Welcome to Yoga: a new way to approach health and well-being. Whether you are seeking help for a particular health problem, or simply in search of some techniques to help improve general feelings of wellness, you will find much in this book that is relevant to you. Before I begin teaching you specific Yoga techniques, however, I invite you to explore with me the idea of wellness from the viewpoint of a Yoga practitioner.

Just as no two people are exactly alike, no two people will express — or achieve — wellness in the same way. I see wellness not just in terms of physical health, but as the enjoyable projection of health, strength, and beauty: the radiant qualities of a balanced individual, with each quality reflecting what is working best for that person in his or her own way. Wellness is a feeling; a pervasive ether. Wellness shines from within when you know you are trying to take good care of yourself. It is a new awareness of your inner strength.

Wellness is an ongoing process. You don't just "get well and forget it," as if it were a goal that you would achieve and then move on to something else. Being well needs the constant support and awareness of everyday practice. In this book you will find the techniques to help yourself recognize and build up the internal support systems that will give you the confidence and balance of that feeling of wellness in everyday life.

Using Yoga techniques for wellness will enhance every aspect of your life. If you have an extremely busy and demanding lifestyle,

Yoga can help you balance the many pressures of work, social life, family, and personal change. If you are an athlete — even a weekend one — Yoga can help you improve the concentration, strength, and flexibility that you need to exercise safely. If you are older, Yoga can help you manage the changes that your body goes through in the course of aging, and give you the confidence and strength to maintain independence in later years.

• *H*ealing Separateness •

Wellness is not a static condition; it involves reaching toward a constantly evolving vision of what we want to be. Even when we have that desire, however, there is a need for support to reach that vision. And when, as most of us do, we visualize ourselves with the mind of a heroic champion, but are working with a "Walter Mitty"-type body, we often experience a split between mind and body. Yoga is unique among fitness programs in that it brings the mind and body together into one unit, healing separateness. Yoga exercises, breathing, and meditation techniques have been used for centuries as a support system which allows those who practice the techniques to reach toward their vision of themselves.

Another problem that sometimes separates the mind from the body is boredom. Most people start out bravely with an exercise routine, but as the novelty wears off, as enthusiasm wanes, and as scheduling problems interfere, the brave new drive to stay well and strong fades away. Yoga, on the other hand, is self-motivating. When you experience the many beneficial effects, you will look forward to your daily practice. Once you begin, you'll find that you actually miss your routine if you don't do it; instead of avoiding it, you will plan for more time to practice. You will never find yourself having to watch television or listen to music while you are doing your exercises, because you won't want to be distracted from what you are doing.

There are three aspects to beginning Yoga practice: exercise (called asana), breathing (called pranayama), and meditation. All three of these affect both mental and physical well-being. Yoga exercises are precise movements of the body and breath that affect all the systems of your body, improving circulation, stabilizing metabolism, and activating the chemicals called endorphins that cause feelings of pleasure. A Yoga routine can be designed to be slow and careful or more vigorous; in either case, your body will never fear Yoga because Yoga is done without strain or force; the stretches, compressions, and balance poses are done with great attention to the needs and capabilities of your own body. Because of this nonviolent approach, you will experience a quietness of mind similar to that of meditation even while exercising.

Yoga breathing exercises strengthen your respiratory system and act as a bridge between the outer and inner worlds. Breathing exercises are your best defense against harmful stress reactions. Depending on which breathing techniques you practice, you can calm yourself or give yourself more energy.

Yoga meditation is a step-by-step process of relaxing the body and quieting the mind. For a few minutes, you simply stop thinking. This brings a tremendous rest and healing to both body and mind.

To attain health and strength, your physical actions must be balanced with your mental being, so they are one unit, not separate. This means that when you are doing anything — eating, talking, walking, seeing, thinking, working — your mind and body are functioning in harmony. You can derive great strength from this joining; you could almost say you would double your strength by pulling your two halves together. This is an exact descrip-

tion of the word "Yoga" which comes from the Sanskrit term "yug," to join. When you practice Yoga, the feeling of separateness begins to heal, and the strong, molded unit of your mind and body starts to operate on its full power.

• The Five Vital Energies •

In the study of Yoga, you will often come across the word "Prana." This word is used to describe the energy system that supports the body and mind. There are five energy centers that make up Prana. The practice of Yoga activates these forces to bring the physical and mental aspects of an individual into balance in wellness.

The first of these energy centers is also called Prana. It operates in the region of the body above the shoulders, through the neck, and all the way to the ends of the hair. The second vital force that Yoga activates in the body is called Apana. It mostly operates out of the region of the navel to the thighs and governs the lower body. Good circulation of blood, essential for health and well-being, is governed by a third vital force of energy called Vyana. Your entire body — from the hair on your head to the bottoms of your feet, wherever blood flows — is affected by Vyana. The fourth vital force is called Samana. Samana means "equalizing." Wholeness, balance, and steadiness result from the activation of Samana and are the strong support for whatever you want to accomplish in this world. The school of Yoga maintains that in order to achieve the enjoyable product of wellness the vital forces of the body must be balanced. Yoga exercises, meditation, and breathing are put together for this very reason.

There is still one vital force I have not mentioned — the most important of these energy centers, known as Udana. It is this force that uplifts us beyond our common everyday consciousness and allows the almost superhuman quality of loss of self — the ability to become that which we are working toward — to appear. This force is seen in those rare moments when a dancer becomes the dance itself; when an athlete achieves something extraordinary; or when a person does something heroic. This force of Udana brings forth intuition and creativity and takes us beyond our normal capabilities. When you experience the clarity of intuition or the exhilaration of creative thought, you will begin to see that this force can be brought forward.

Udana is the most neglected vital source in our bodies and minds, perhaps because little is known in the everyday world about how it works. In the body, it governs the spinal column and a nerve called shushumna that runs the length of the spine up into the brain. In books on Yoga, the power in this nerve is often described as kundalini. Some people mistakenly try to "awaken" this kundalini force by practicing intense breathing and physical exercises without the proper preparation of exercise, correct diet, and regular practice; this can lead to great upset in the body and mind. The Yoga practices of exercise, breathing, and meditation described in this book will help balance your body and mind so that the strength of this nerve in the spine awakens correctly and safely.

Unlike the other vital energies, which work with the force of gravity, Udana works the opposite way. It moves up in the body, bringing about a great feeling of lightness and flexibility — like flying without a parachute. Its greatest quality is detachment, and when it is functioning well, you have the opportunity to experience exquisitely clear perception.

Whatever your present state of health, the techniques described in this book will help you achieve the balance and strength of all the body's energies. With daily practice, you will feel the beneficial effects very soon. As these energy centers begin to function, your eyes will twinkle, your heart will become stronger, your walk will become straighter, and your mind will become more creative and balanced.

I wish you the best of success in your practice of Yoga for inner strength, shining health, and vibrant well-being.

Wellness and Ethics

When practicing Yoga under the direction of a competent teacher, the student is constantly reminded to follow ethical behavior in all aspects of life. Ethical conduct helps to protect you from upset and illness. When you adhere to ethical behavior, your strength is not depleted by debilitating fear or guilt, and you avoid doing things that harm your body and mind.

The practice of ethics in Yoga has a different meaning from that of a religious orientation. Many people mistake Yoga for a religious practice because of the widespread belief that Yoga is an offshoot of Hinduism. Actually, Yoga comes from a much older tradition based not on any religious creeds or beliefs but purely on individual experience. In Yoga, ethics are practiced for the benefit of the individual, whereas in religion they are often taught as moral rules that primarily benefit society. It is true that the constant practice of ethical behavior will eventually affect all of your relationships. But as a Yoga student, your ethical conduct has to do first and foremost with yourself. The idea is to get yourself and your life in order first before you take on the rest of the world. This is the real meaning of the old adage, "Charity begins at home."

There are ten specific ethical guidelines in Yoga: nonviolence, not lying, not stealing, no casual sex, non-hoarding, purity, contentment, tolerance, study, and remembrance. Checking daily on these points as they pertain to your actions and thoughts will show you a clear path of behavior that will bring balance and health into your life. When you see the positive effects that come from practicing this discipline, you will practice it quite happily. Sometimes the practice of ethics is viewed as something difficult or painful. In Yoga, ethics are used only to clarify and purify the life of the individual. They serve the individual in every way, and because of their valuable support, the Yoga student finds them not only enjoyable but indispensable.

In ancient times, Yoga students would present themselves to a teacher only after long periods of mental and physical purification that involved the mastery of these ethical concepts. The way someone begins to practice Yoga seems to be very different now, but in fact it is much the same. Whether you choose to practice Yoga intensively or simply to learn some techniques for health, relaxation, and peace of mind, you can achieve this same kind of purification and balance in your life by regular practice of ethics, guiding yourself by yourself. They will help you and give you support in your search for health and the wonderful feeling of wellness.

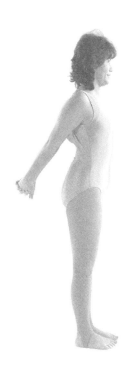

• *W*hat is Yoga? •

Yoga is a system of exercise, breathing, and meditation techniques designed for health and self-awareness. Most people in the United States are more familiar with the physical aspects of Yoga: the poses or movements that build flexibility, balance, and strength. These exercises were originally developed in order to achieve maximum health in the shortest time and in the smallest space possible; thus, they are very efficient techniques. Meditation in Yoga involves simply stopping all thought for a period of time. This practice eventually brings steadiness, self-awareness, and the realization of an inner source of strength, power, and creativity that supports you in everything you do.

Yoga is not a cure-all for disease; however, the techniques of Yoga can help relieve symptoms, reinforce lifestyle changes, build strength and flexibility, reduce pain, and improve your quality of life. Most importantly, Yoga can help you prevent serious disease by instilling positive, healthy fitness habits and attitudes.

• *H*ow to Use This Book •

In this book we have designed routines specific to 15 different health problems; these are presented in Chapters 2 through 16. The current chapter (Chapter 1) presents a "Basic Routine" comprised of several exercises that are so broadly effective that we recommend

them for everyone, including a series of warmups and complete instructions for breathing techniques, relaxation and meditation procedures, and the "I Love You" meditation technique. We recommend that you start by reviewing the techniques in this chapter; then turn to the chapter on the health problem that concerns you to find special instructions and additional techniques that are particularly helpful for that problem.

Your daily routine will take between 30 and 45 minutes every day. If you are not strong enough to do the full routine, do at least three exercises every day and a few minutes of meditation. Here's how to put your routine together:

Begin with breathing exercises (pp. 24-26)

Continue with warmup exercises (pp. 16-20)

Add the essential Yoga exercises (pp. 21-24)

Go to the chapter in the book that describes your particular health problem and do at least three of the exercises in that section

End with relaxation and meditation (pp. 26-27)

Doing the routine all at once will help you achieve a quieter and more restful meditation, but if your schedule doesn't allow enough time all at once, you can split up the routine and do warmups and exercises at one time of day, breathing and meditation at another. For the best continuity as you practice the exercises, do the standing ones first, then the floor exercises, so each exercise flows smoothly into the next. The exercises in each chapter are arranged accordingly.

The techniques in this chapter can be used as a complete maintenance routine for days when time is particularly short.

• Cautions and Hints •

Always Check with Your Physician

We highly recommend that you obtain your physician's approval before beginning any of the routines in this book. Only a professional familiar with your current medical condition and history will be able to help you judge which techniques you should and should not do.

Yoga and Children

Because of the effect of Yoga exercises on the glandular system, Yoga exercise is not recommended for persons under 16 years of age. Until the age of 16, the body's glandular system is still developing, and it is possible that some Yoga exercises will overstimulate the system and disrupt the natural developmental process.

If they wish, young people who are interested in Yoga may practice meditation happily and successfully. The "I Love You" meditation technique is especially recommended for increasing self-esteem and self-confidence.

Women's Issues

Menstruation.   During the days of heaviest flow, you should not do the exercise portion of your routine; Yoga exercises put pressure on glands and organs that could result in extremely heavy bleeding, or upset to the nervous system. Breathing and meditation, however, are always helpful.

Pregnancy.   During your first trimester, breathing and meditation may be practiced every day as often as you wish. Yoga exercises, however, should not be done during this period. After the first trimester, with your physician's permission, you may do a modified routine of exercise. See our other beginning books (listed in Resources) for special routines for pregnancy.

• Your Yoga Environment •

Clothing

Wear clothes that are loose and comfortable, or stretchy. Stay warm — especially during meditation. Exercising in bare feet is best, but slip on a pair of socks before you go into meditation.

Space and Equipment

Choose a small blanket, beach towel, or mat to use only for Yoga practice. You will also need several small cushions for the seated breathing exercises and another blanket or shawl to cover yourself during meditation as protection against chill. Practice in a quiet, draft-free room where you won't be disturbed. Make sure pets are in another room, and turn off your telephone during meditation to protect yourself from disturbance.

Time of Day

For best results, practice Yoga at the same time each day. If your schedule doesn't allow that, practice when you can fit it in, but try to do something every day; even a few minutes a day will keep the momentum of Yoga practice alive and provide faster results.

Food, Caffeine, Alcohol, Medication

Don't exercise immediately after a large meal; wait an hour or two. The same rule applies to caffeine. Never practice Yoga under the influence of alcohol or recreational drugs. If you are taking medication that causes you to feel drowsy, wait until the effect has lessened before practicing your daily routine, and check with your doctor if you take such medication regularly.

• *H*ow to Practice Yoga Excercises •

Read First

For best results, read the instructions thoroughly and imagine yourself doing the exercise before you actually try it. This way you will learn the movements faster, and you won't have to keep referring to the book as you move.

Avoid Pain

Yoga exercise should not hurt. Never stretch to the point of pain, and never bounce or jerk in any of the movements. Treat your body as your friend, not your enemy.

Breathe as Instructed

Each Yoga exercise has a particular breathing pattern. It is very important to follow the instructions about breath exactly, because the proper movement of the breath is an important part of what makes the exercise work. Always breathe through your nose.

Move Slowly

Think about each movement as you do it. All Yoga movements are slow, controlled, and done with controlled breathing. Pay attention to the proper positioning of your hands and eyes, and to the relaxation of any muscles that you are not using for the exercise.

Repetitions

Most exercises call for only three repetitions. This is because Yoga exercises are so efficient that you do not need to do any more repetitions to achieve the desired effect.

Holding

Most exercises involve a brief hold when the breath is in or out, instructing you to hold to a count of three. This does not mean a strict three-second count; it can and should be a faster count in the beginning as you build strength. This brief hold increases the effectiveness of the exercise.

How to Avoid Injury

All Yoga exercises should be done slowly and deliberately so you always know how your body is feeling. As you exercise, think about what you are doing. Be aware of your breath, the position of your hands and feet, and any stiffness in your spine. Pay attention to the messages your body sends you through your muscles, nerves, and joints — especially those that indicate you may be pushing too much! It is always a good idea to do an exercise at half capacity when you are first learning it to avoid straining. Also, if you read the instructions through completely, you won't find yourself holding a position longer than you should because you forgot what to do next and had to consult your book.

When practicing Yoga exercises for the first time, you may notice a slight stiffness, especially in the back of your legs, if you are not used to stretching. In Yoga you should stretch only as far as you can without pain, and you should never bounce or jerk. The benefit of stretching a muscle comes from holding it in a relaxed position. In the Sun Poses, for example, you bend forward as you breathe out, and then hold the position and your breath for a count of three. During that brief holding time, try to relax every muscle that is not being used for the exercise; if you can do this, you will notice that your muscles elongate a bit more as they relax. Never hold a position longer than recommended. Yoga exercises are designed to be so efficient that they give you maximum benefit for minimum time and effort.

• *W*armup Exercises •

Warming up your body is a way to find out how you feel. Listen to your body's messages about muscle tension or pain. The warmups are gentle movements that begin to get your circulation moving, test the range of motion in your joints, and begin to stretch the major muscle groups. Most of these exercises can be done seated in a chair or even in bed.

Shoulder Roll. *Loosens shoulder joints and upper back muscles.* Keeping your arms and hands loose at your sides, lift your shoulders (**A**) and roll them forward, down, back, and up in a smooth circle. Continue rolling forward three or four times; then reverse and roll back, down, forward, and up several times. Keep arms and hands loose. Breathe normally. The purpose of this exercise is to loosen the muscles of the upper back and shoulders, where a lot of tension is held, especially at the end of the day. If you work at a desk much of the day, do this exercise several times a day to keep from building up tension in your upper back and neck.

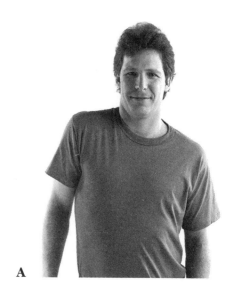

A

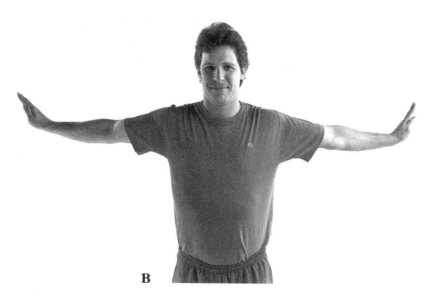

B

Arm Circles. *Increases circulation; strengthens back and shoulders; improves range of motion of shoulders; limbers upper back, chest, and midback muscles.* Hold your arms straight out to the sides with elbows straight and flex your hands back toward your face, fingers together (**B**). Maintaining that position, slowly rotate your arms forward in large circles — as large as possible, so you exercise the full range of motion of your shoulder joints. Keep the fingers stretched back. Do three or four large circles in each direction, then do a few smaller circles in each direction. Let your arms relax, and shake them out. Breathe normally throughout this exercise.

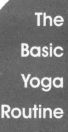

The Basic Yoga Routine

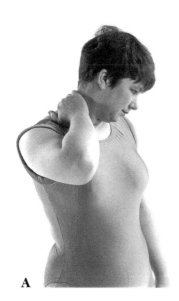

A

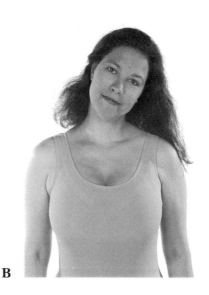

B

Neck Stretch. *Releases tension in upper back and neck.* Gently bend your head down and to the right without bending your upper back, so your chin comes down toward your collarbone while looking to the right as far as you can. Put your left hand up to the left side of your neck to feel the muscles stretching (**A**). Hold for a few seconds, breathing normally. Now bring your head back up straight and bend down and toward the left. Push your chin down toward your collarbone while looking to the left as far as you can. Put your right hand on the right side of your neck and feel the muscles stretching tight. Relax. Massage your neck with both hands (see p. 55).

Next, gently tilt your head to the left (**B**), bring it back up straight, and tilt down toward the right. [Repeat twice more] Now look straight ahead and slowly turn your head to look over your left shoulder. Slowly turn back and all the way over to the right shoulder. [Repeat twice more]

If these movements feel comfortable, try a gentle rotation: Slowly lower your right ear toward your right shoulder, next drop your chin toward your chest, then gently bring your left ear toward your left shoulder, and slowly bring your head up straight. All of these variations can be done with hands supporting the neck as in (**A**). [3 each direction]

Elbow Twist. *Limbers spine; improves respiration and posture.* Stand with your feet several inches apart. Extend your arms, horizontally, bending them at the elbow, and place one hand on top of the other. Breathe in, straightening your spine, and breathe out as you twist slowly around to one side, leading with one elbow (**C**). Twist as far around as you can, feeling the stretch all along your spine from your tailbone to the back of your neck. Stretch your eyes and facial muscles by looking back over your shoulder as far as possible. Breathe in and return to the front, then breathe out and twist to the opposite side. [3 each direction, alternating]

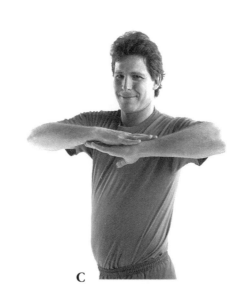

C

Easy Balance. *Improves respiration; oxygenates blood; strengthens ankles and calves; improves balance.* Breathe out, arms at your sides. Staring at one spot to help maintain balance, breathe in completely, stretch up on your toes, and press your fists into your diaphragm (**A**). (Be sure you are not pressing into your rib cage, but directly below it.) Hold for a count of three. Breathe out and relax, lowering your arms and heels. [3 repetitions]

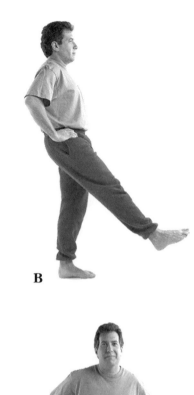

B

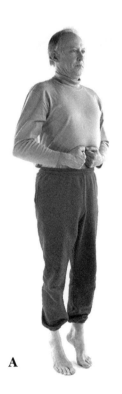

A

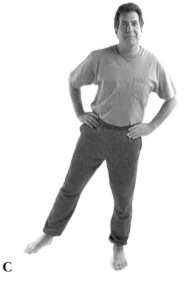

C

Leg Lifts. *Limbers hip joints; strengthens legs; improves balance.* Put both hands on your hips. Lift your left leg toward the front (**B**), with the toes pulled back toward your face and both knees straight. Lower the leg. Repeat twice more. Now lift it to the side (**C**), and lower. Repeat twice more. Lift it to the back (**D**), keeping your knee straight, then lower. Repeat twice more. Breathe normally throughout this exercise. [3 forward, side, and back, each leg]

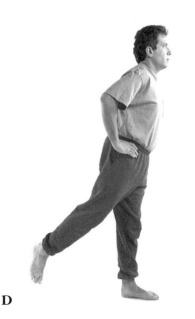

D

Full Bend and Hold. *Releases tension in the upper back and neck; helps to reduce a large stomach.* Stand straight, arms at your sides. Breathe out completely through your nose, then breathe in as you lift your arms up, out to the sides, and back as far as you can without straining (**A**). Hold for a count of three, then breathe out and bend forward, leading with your arms. When you are as far forward as possible (keeping your knees straight), relax your arms and head and let them hang (**B**). Hold for a count of three, then come back up, breathing in and raising your arms up, out, and to the sides as before. Repeat twice more.

After your third repetition, breathe out and come forward once again but let your arms relax toward the floor. If you can reach the floor comfortably, let your fingers curl slightly. Just go limp and relax, let your head hang so your neck stretches, and relax your breath. Hold for several seconds, then slowly stand up. If your lower back is tight, don't hold as long.

Full Bend Variation. *Improves posture; limbers shoulder joints and upper back vertebrae; improves respiration.* Clasp your hands behind your back and straighten your arms (**C**). If you can, lock your elbows as shown and press your palms together so your shoulder blades are squeezed together. Breathe in, standing straight, then breathe out and bend forward, keeping your arms pulled back and away from your body (**D**). Keep knees straight. Breathe in and straighten back to your starting position. If it is difficult to sustain the arms-locked position for all three repetitions, relax your arms, shake them out, and gently roll your head back and forth between each sequence. [3 repetitions]

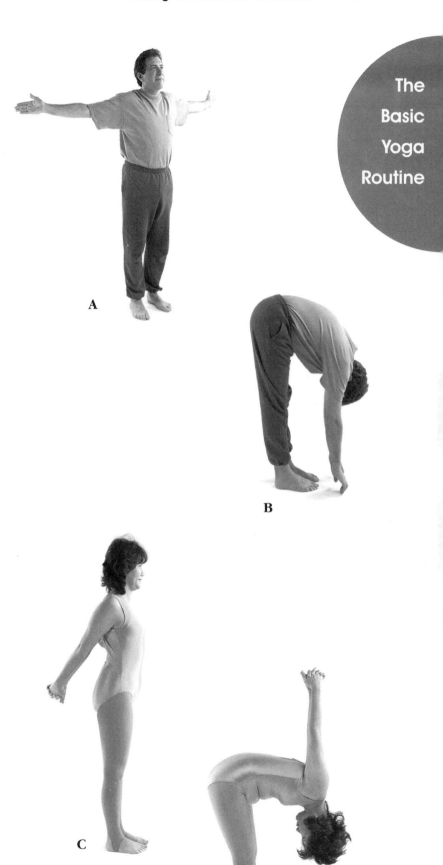

The
Basic
Yoga
Routine

A

B

C

D

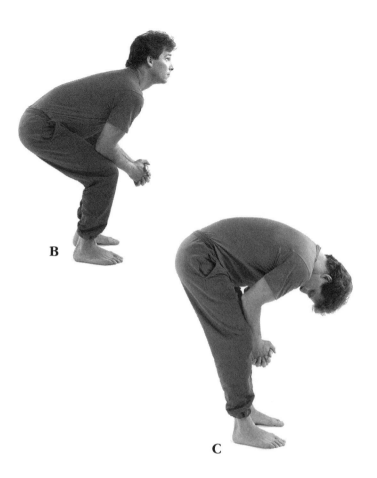

B

C

Standing Twist. *Same benefits as Standing Reach, plus improves flexibility of spine, and strengthens legs and feet.* Breathe in and reach up, come up on your toes, press your palms together, hold the breath in and twist to one side (**A**). Stare at one spot for balance. Hold for a count of three, then turn back forward and relax. [3 times each direction]

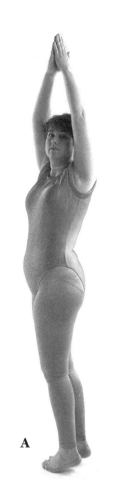

A

Lazy Stretch. *Stretches back of legs and lower back; strengthens ankles and calves; improves respiration.* Stand with feet shoulder width apart. Bend your knees and rest your forearms on your knees with hands clasped. Breathe in and look up, arching your back slightly (**B**). Breathe out and straighten your legs while keeping your forearms on your knees (**C**). Tuck your chin toward your chest. [3 repetitions]

Standing Reach. *Improves breathing, posture, and balance.* Breathe out completely, arms at your sides. Breathe in and reach up over your head, press your palms together, stretch up (**D**), hold for a count of three, then breathe out and lower. [3 repetitions]

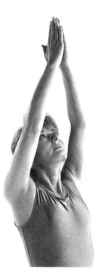

D

• *T*he Essential Yoga Exercises •

Standing Sun Pose. *Improves function-ing of digestive and circulatory systems; exer-cises heart and lungs; limbers and strengthens legs and back.* Stand with feet parallel. Breathe out completely. Start to breathe in and raise your arms in a circle to the sides (**A**) and over your head, palms to-gether (**D,** previous page). Your breath should be all the way in. Look up at your hands. Now breathe out as you bend forward from the waist, keeping your back as straight as you can for as long as possible (**B**). Keep your head between your arms. Grasp your an-kles, calves, or knees with both hands (get a good, firm grip) and bend your elbows slightly to pull your upper body toward your legs (**C**). Your breath should now be com-pletely out. Keep your knees straight and tuck your chin. Hold for a count of three.

Important: If you can't bend your elbows, you're grasping too far down your legs. Move your grip higher so you can bend your el-bows; otherwise, you'll be pulling with your back muscles, which could strain your back. Be sure to use your arms to pull yourself down.

After holding for a count of three with your breath out, release your legs and slowly come back up to a standing position, breath-ing in as you bring your arms out to the sides and up in a circular motion. Stretch and look up with palms together, then breathe out and lower your arms to your sides in a final circle. Always move your arms in as wide a circle as you can in order to increase the expansion of the chest. [3 repetitions]

The
Basic
Yoga
Routine

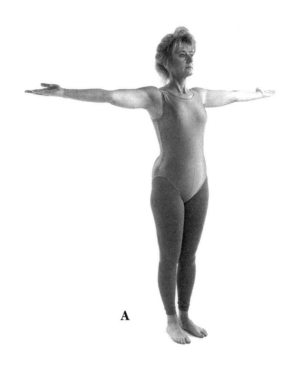

A

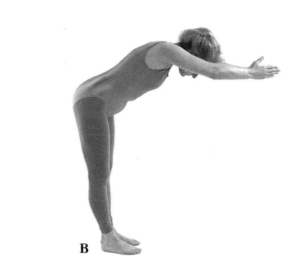

B

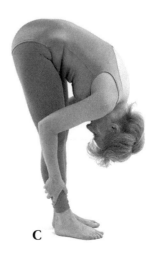

C

Seated Sun Pose.   *Stretches back of legs; limbers and strengthens lower back; massages internal organs.* Sit straight with both legs stretched in front, toes pulled back toward your face, arms at your sides. Breathe in as you lift your arms to the sides (**A**) and overhead (**B**). Look up and stretch, elongating your spine. Then breathe out and bend forward over your legs, tucking your chin. Grasp your ankles or calves with both hands (**C**) (or, if you can reach your toes comfortably, grasp the toes as shown in **D**). Bend your arms and pull gently. Hold for a count of three. Then release, breathe in and bring your arms in another circle to the sides and overhead. Look up. Breathe out and lower your arms to your sides. [3 repetitions]

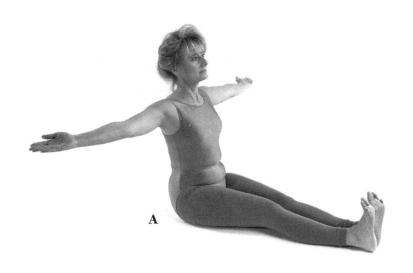

A

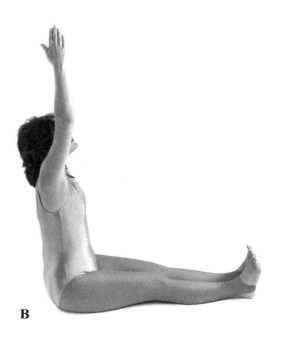

B

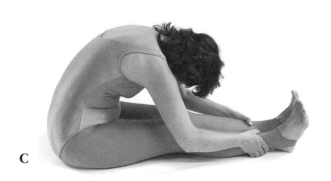

C

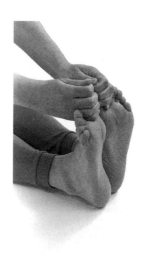

D

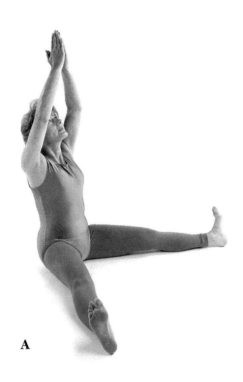

A

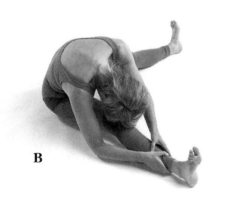

B

Tortoise Stretch.   *Improves circulation to pelvic region; stretches nerves and muscles in legs and ankles; limbers lower back; helps prevent prostate problems.* Sit with legs separated as far as possible. Pull your feet back toward your face, lean back on your hands, lift your hips slightly and push your pelvis forward. Then sit straight, rest your hands on your legs, and point your toes. Hold for a few seconds. Repeat twice more.

Now, with feet pulled back again, breathe in and raise your arms in a circle over your head. Look up (**A**). Now breathe out and bend toward your left leg. Grasp the ankle or calf of your leg with both hands and bend your elbows slightly, pulling your upper body gently toward your leg (**B**). Tuck your chin and keep your knees straight. (If you can reach your toes comfortably and still bend your arms, wrap your left hand around the big toe and grasp the arch of your foot with your right hand.) Your breath should be completely out. Hold for a count of three, then breathe in as you raise your arms in a circular motion overhead, look up, then breathe out and lower your arms over your right leg. [3 each side]

Now lean forward between your legs as far as you can without strain, supporting yourself with arms stretched forward on the floor (**C**), and just rest, breathing normally, for a few seconds.

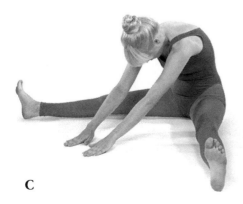

C

Baby Pose.   *Limbers and relaxes lower back; improves circulation to the brain and pelvic region; improves reproductive and digestive systems functioning; improves respiration; reduces large stomach.* Sit on your feet with knees together. Slowly bend forward so your head touches the floor (**A**). Let your arms rest at your sides with your elbows bent so they rest on the floor. This will relax your shoulders and neck. Your head can rest on the forehead or bridge of the nose. Settle yourself into the most comfortable position you can find. Let your breath relax, and hold for at least a minute. If this position is not comfortable, try resting your head on folded arms (**B**); if that is still too uncomfortable, use this position as an exercise, hold it for only a few seconds, then lie down on your back to rest.

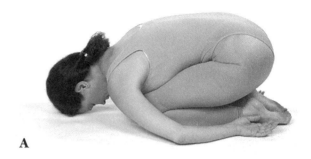

A

• *B*reathing Techniques •

Your seated position.   A comfortable seated position is essential for breathing techniques. Take time to establish a comfortable seat, whether on the floor or on the edge of a chair. If you are sitting on the floor, place a few cushions under your hips (**C**); this will tilt your pelvis slightly forward so that your lower back and stomach can relax. If you try to sit without support under your hips, you won't be able to breathe easily. If your knees aren't limber enough so that they rest below your hips in this position, add cushions or sit on the edge of a chair with feet tucked under slightly (don't lean back) (**D**). You can also try straddling a pile of cushions.

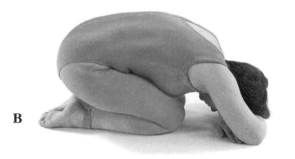

B

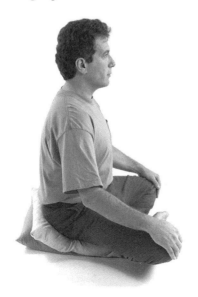

C

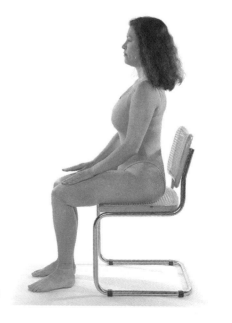

D

Always breathe through the nose. As you breathe, close your throat very slightly so that you hear a steamlike sound as you breathe in and out. Concentrating on this sound will help you concentrate on the breath and will draw your mind inward.

When to practice breathing. In the beginning, practice breathing at the beginning of your routine to help get you in the mood to practice and to help turn your mind away from external thoughts. If you wish, you can also do a few breath cycles just prior to meditation. You can also use the breathing exercises — particularly the Complete Breath — any time of day to help quiet physical responses to stress: rapid heartbeat and breathing, tense muscles, and so on.

Belly Breath. *Improves respiration; strengthens diaphragm and other respiratory muscles.* Place your hands loosely on your belly below your navel. Breathe in through your nose and relax your belly as you imagine that you are filling your belly with air, expanding it and pushing your hands outward (**A**). This movement will relax all your internal organs and cause the diaphragm to drop to its fullest extent, allowing the air to reach the bottom section of your lungs. Breathe out now, through your nose, and slowly, consciously, contract your belly muscles, pushing in with your hands until all the air is out (**B**). Repeat several times. Remember: as you inhale the belly expands outward; as you exhale the belly contracts inward.

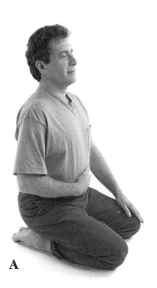

A

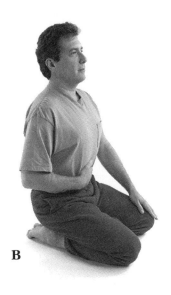

B

Complete Breath. *Stretches and strengthens all the muscles of the chest, rib cage, and stomach; helps reduce harmful stress reactions.* The Complete Breath starts just like the Belly Breath, above, but continues the expansion into the ribs and chest as well, stretching and strengthening all of the respiratory muscles. Start by placing your hands on your belly. Inhale and push your belly forward, expanding it; exhale and tighten your belly muscles, pushing the air out. Notice that when you inhale, as you relax and push your belly forward, you get a slight tilt in your lower back as well.

Now place your hands higher so you can feel your ribs. Your fingertips should be just touching. Inhale and expand the ribs, noticing that your fingers are pulled apart slightly; exhale and contract your ribs, noticing your fingers touching again.

Finally, move on to expand the chest. After you've expanded your belly and your ribs, your lungs will be nearly full. At the top of the inhalation, expand the top of your chest just slightly to get the last of the air in; your shoulders will naturally lift just a little. Don't strain.

The exhalation is done in reverse: As you begin to exhale, relax your shoulders and chest first, then the ribs, then tighten the belly. Don't hold your breath in or out; make the transition smooth. Try to breathe for about the same length of time both ways, and always breathe through your nose.

Concentrate on that steamlike sound of the breath in the back of your throat. Breathe in from the bottom up; breathe out from the top down. At first, you'll be using all your attention just to learn the pattern of the breath. After you've been practicing for a while, your mind may start to drift while you're breathing; gently bring your attention back to the sound of the breath.

At first, practice 5 or more repetitions of the Complete Breath every day in a seated position. Then, try practicing the breath technique whenever you think of it — at the office, in the car, while you're waiting in line at the grocer — and notice how you feel while you're breathing. Does the breath change how you feel?

• *R*elaxation and Meditation •

For best results in meditation, lie on your back on your mat or blanket on the floor or in bed (**A,** next page). Don't put a pillow under your head. (If you are unable to lie on your back, you can sit in a recliner chair or some other chair that keeps your back straight yet relaxed; it is most important in meditation that your spine be straight.) If your lower back is tense, place a few pillows under your knees.

Wear socks and throw a blanket or shawl over you so you don't get chilled; your body temperature naturally will drop as you relax and become quiet. Make sure your pets are in another room so they won't disturb you. Turn your telephone off, and ask your family not to interrupt you during these few minutes. Protect yourself as much as possible from sharp noises while you are quiet and still in meditation.

Begin with a complete relaxation procedure that will take about 5 minutes. (If you use our Complete Relaxation and Meditation audiotape, the tape will talk you through this sequence — see Resources.) Go through the following sequence, taking your time visualizing and relaxing each muscle and bone and

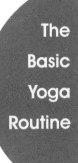

joint of your body. Let your breath relax into a natural pattern.

Start by closing your eyes. Think about your forehead; relax it, smooth out any lines, any tension. Now relax your eyes, without moving them. Think about how they look, and relax all the muscles around your eyes. Continue to relax your face, including your teeth, tongue, and lips. Relax the corners of your mouth, and the hinges of your jaw.

Relax your neck and shoulders. Visualize each part of your body and relax it, spending several seconds on each part. Relax your arms, elbows, wrists, and hands.

Visualize your heart, take a deep breath, and sigh the breath out, relaxing your heart. Think about your lungs, take another breath, and breathe out, relaxing your lungs. Then let your breath go back to normal.

Continue moving down your body, relaxing your hips, the long bones in your thighs, your knees, ankles, and feet. Then relax the back of your legs. Now visualize your spine. Relax your tailbone, then move up your spine, relaxing each bone in your lower back, mid-

back, and shoulder blades. Relax the back of your neck, and the bones of your skull. Then visualize your brain and imagine it floating inside your skull.

Now bring your attention back to your forehead. Think of the sound "om" (pronounced "ohm"). This sound is a mantram, a word that is believed by Yogis to have a particular effect on the mind. This word "om" has been used by Yoga practitioners for thousands of years to represent the stillness of meditation. Repeat it several times to yourself. Then just think nothing. Don't force yourself to be quiet; just rest and gently try to stop all inner conversation. Think nothing. See how long you can remain still before another thought creeps in. As soon as you notice yourself thinking, gently let the thought go and think nothing again.

After 10 to 15 minutes, slowly move your fingers and toes, take a deep breath, stretch, and lie quietly for a minute or so observing how you feel. Never leap right up out of meditation. Come out slowly. Then go about your day with renewed energy and happiness.

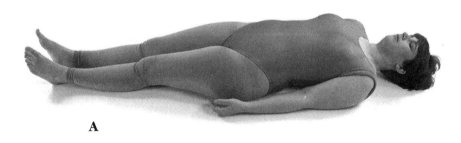

A

• *T*he "I Love You" Meditation Technique •

A vital quality for anyone is self-confidence — especially if you're not feeling well. The "I Love You" meditation technique, practiced regularly, will help. This technique should be done as a complement to — rather than as a substitute for — daily meditation as described above. (For an audio- or videotape of this technique, see Resources.)

Research has shown that positive feelings have very beneficial effects on the body's immune system, contributing to better health and faster recovery from stress. The "I Love You" technique builds self-esteem and removes unseen fear. It will also improve your relationships because you will find that your view of yourself doesn't depend on anyone else's opinion. It has a soothing, calming effect that will help you rest and sleep better than ever before.

Start with the Laughasan exercise (below): Lie on your back and start pumping your legs as if you were riding a bicycle. Move your arms, too, and start to laugh. Pump your arms and legs as vigorously as you can and laugh out loud for at least 30 seconds. Then relax and settle into your relaxation position.

Lie on your back comfortably, without a pillow under your head, on your bed or the floor, or in a recliner chair that keeps your back straight. Cover yourself with a blanket or shawl. Make sure your pets are in another room and that your telephone is turned off. Let your arms rest at your sides with the palms up, a very vulnerable position, like a baby's hands. Press your back slightly toward the floor, then release and relax. Pull your chin down a little toward your chest without straining, to stretch the cords in the back of the neck that will allow more movement of the feeling that is going to affect the brain. Your arms should be close to your body and

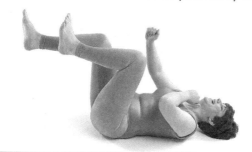

your legs together. If your lower back is tense, place a few pillows under your knees.

Now bring your attention to your forehead and breathe in, saying "I love you" to yourself as you breathe in. Breathe out and say "I love you." Repeat this several times, breathing in "I love you" and breathing out "I love you." Now breathe in and hold for a moment. Imagine the feeling "I love you" spreading throughout your brain, warm and wet, perfumed, beautiful — like everything you think of as lovely. Breathe out saying "I love you."

Now totally relax. Let your breath do what it wants. And just hold that feeling. In your own way now, continue to say "I love you" on your breath: Breathe in "I love you" and breathe out "I love you."

Now think to yourself: Whom do I love? Breathe in. Hold your breath. Whom do you love? Breathe out and say "I love you." Whom do I love? Breathe in: Who loves me? Hold your breath. Now think to yourself: "My breath loves me." The breath is inside you. It loves you. Breathe out. "My breath loves me." Breathe in — "I'm holding my breath — it loves me." Breathe out — "I have released my breath — It still loves me." Again: take a deep breath, always through your nose. Breathe in: "My breath loves me." Breathe out: "My breath is gone now but it still loves me."

Now relax completely. Visualize the inside of your head and your body. Think of this love that's there with your breath. It's bringing oxygen into your body and it's flowing through your veins and heart and every part of you because you can't live without your breath. Visualize this loving thing that is inside your body, and see if there are blocks anywhere keeping it from moving where it wants to go. Visualize this feeling removing any kind of block or constriction. It's going to move easily and sweetly.

Bring it to your forehead. Think "I love you" — my breath is in my forehead. Relax your forehead so that that breath of love permeates your whole forehead. Now think of your eyes. This quality of the breath of love comes into your eyes. You can feel a slight wind. Your eyes are just looking at this magnificent thing. Now relax your eyes and let the breath of love simply swim out into your eyes. Relax the rest of your face like this. Your nose should especially feel this breath of love because it breathes for you. Every time you breathe in, breathe "I love you." Every time you breathe out, breathe "I love you." Thank your nose for working; it's the tool for this love to come into your body. Open the channels in your face that would flow freely to make your face melt with love. Let your mouth hang and relax; think "That breath is coming into my mouth all the time whether I pay any attention to it or not. And it's going out all the time. And it loves me. It comes there because it loves me, and I love it."

Now relax your throat the same way. Think of this breath that's bringing all this beautiful blood into your system. Everything is very clear. Let your neck relax now so you have no constriction that will stop it from moving. Now the love comes in — relax. Now the love goes out — relax. Now drop your collarbone toward the floor and say "I love you." Let the ends of your shoulders drop toward the floor. Do the same thing with your arms; let them relax toward the floor because they are fully supported by this breath of love. You're looking at your elbows in your mind's eye. Look at your elbow and love it. Your elbow loves you. Rest your arms in love. Relax your wrists. Let your hands be totally relaxed in love. You're vulnerable. You don't care. You can't lose it. It comes in and it goes out. Relax your fingers. Say "I love you" to your fingers.

Now go to your chest. This time you are going to be aware that you are taking in that breath. You're taking a breath in: "I love you." It's going to your heart. Breathe it out. "I'm losing you; I still love you." Same with the lungs. Breathe in: "I love you." Breathe out: "I love you." Now relax your whole chest. Let it breathe as it wants to. But you then are going to become aware that this is love. You're not making it happen. It's happening because it loves you.

Now breathe in and think of your stomach. Breathe out: "I love you." Relax your stomach. Think of your abdomen. Relax your abdomen: "I love you. I love you the way you are." Now relax. Relax your hip joints. Actually feel the breath of love move through the hip joint. Warm, liquid, lubricating, beautiful — it's like perfect balance and poise. Now say "I love you" to your hips and relax them. Let the large bones in the top of the legs get very flat toward the floor; you don't have to hold them up with any nerves. You love them. They love you. You can't lose love. Relax your legs — in love. Let your legs totally relax, because love is there. Think about your legs: "I love you." Relax them. "You don't have to be afraid; I love you." Relax your knees and ankles and think "I love you." Now relax your feet. Your feet are completely supported in love. Think to your feet "I love you." Relax your feet.

Now picture yourself just simply floating; completely supported on this thing, this love. Bring your mind back up to the back of your hips and the base of your spine. Just open it up like a flower. Say "I love you." Don't fight it. Let it flow easily. Just let it go, smooth and quiet. Relax the back of your shoulder blades. Let your back get soft. Take away any effort because love is supporting you. "I love you, back." Now the back of your neck drops a little bit. And think to yourself, "I love you. I love you." Come back up to your head now. Picture yourself in your hair. Feel love oozing out through your hair. "I love you. It's what makes my hair. It makes my brain."

Breathe in and think love. Breathe out — you think love goes, but it doesn't. It comes right back. Relax your brain. Think of it floating in a puddle of this love, like a fluid. It's so happy there. Like a baby happily playing in a bathtub full of suds. Now make it quiet. Totally quiet. And say "I love you." Then bring your mind to your forehead and think nothing. If you feel any other thought coming in, make sure that it says "I love you." Transpose any thought to "I love you" and go back to thinking nothing. Think nothing as long as you can. Stop talking to yourself altogether. Become silent internally.

Rest quietly like this for about ten minutes, then slowly stretch, take a deep breath and let it out, and think about how you feel. Rest on your side or stomach for a few minutes enjoying the feeling before you get up. Move slowly back into your normal attitudes and lifestyle.

• *T*he Importance of a Proper Diet •

Sometimes, when we don't feel at our best, we don't feel much like eating — let alone going to the effort of shopping for and preparing nutritious meals. But a balanced, nutritious diet can be a very good defense against illness as well as a support to help you to recover faster. Most of the chapters in this book contain some specific dietary suggestions for the different physical conditions described. If you are interested in more complete information about how to create and maintain a healthy diet, there are many excellent books and periodicals available (see Appendix B, Further Reading).

Healthy Choices

Changing your diet should be done slowly and informatively; an abrupt change in how you eat can cause almost as much stress on your body as eating poorly. If you are not sure about whether your diet is adequate or not, consult a reputable nutritionist or a good book on general nutrition. If you are like most people, your diet will probably be low in fresh fruits and vegetables and whole grains, approximately adequate in protein, and too high in fat and sugar.

When you are not feeling well, your need for nutrients increases. Similarly, if you smoke, drink alcohol several times a week, or drink a lot of coffee, tea, or other caffeinated beverages every day, your need for nutrients increases. Some medications also deplete your body, as do fluorescent lights, stress, and environmental pollution. Overly processed foods and those with added chemicals — especially artificial flavors and colors — can often cause allergic reactions.

All these factors make it essential to create a diet that you can be sure contains the nutrients your body needs to get well and stay well. Most of my students have discovered that supplementing a balanced diet with essential vitamins and minerals helps ensure that their bodies are getting enough of what they need for good health and repair.

Should You Become a Vegetarian?

You certainly don't need to become a vegetarian to practice beginning Yoga techniques or to become well, but modern medicine is recognizing the healthful aspects of a balanced vegetarian diet. The recent "Mediterranean Diet" craze, though not strictly vegetarian, emphasizes fresh fruits and vegetables and whole grains; when meat is included, it is fish or poultry in small amounts. I have been a vegetarian for over 40 years, and although my main reason for following this type of diet has mostly to do with my desire to follow the ethical guidelines of nonviolence in my Yoga practice, I have also found that this type of diet has brought me luminous health, energy, and well-being. I do not advocate the extreme macrobiotic diet — I have seen people become quite ill from it — but rather a balanced vegetarian diet that includes low-fat dairy, occasional eggs, and plenty of whole grains, fresh vegetables, and fruit.

If you decide to try this type of diet, spend a few weeks counting protein grams every day to be sure you are getting enough. Your best protein sources are low-fat dairy products, tofu, legumes, and whole grains. You can find charts for the protein content of common foods in many of the books listed in Appendix B.

Breathing Disorders and Diet: A Personal Story

My oldest son was born with bronchial asthma. It was a terrifying time for me to see him fight for breath, especially in the night. I was fortunate to make the acquaintance of Adelle Davis, a great nutritionist of her time, when both of us were speaking at a convention. She told me how to help my son with diet and nutritional supplementation. I followed her instructions with great care and my boy improved remarkably. (See Appendix B for a listing of some of Davis's books.)

The hardest part of Adelle's recommended diet was removing coal tar products (the top offenders are artificial flavor and color) from our daily diet. Aspirin, some other medications, and (in those days) margarine were all affected. Bakery products had to be checked carefully for "baker's yellow." Usually I found only one fool-proof solution — I had to make it myself! I started on a long program that continues even today: my family loved homemade breads, ice cream, fresh fruits and vegetables, and homemade soups. I found a wonderful resource in the fresh, wholesome products sold by Walnut Acres in Pennsylvania (see Appendix B); their whole-wheat and spinach pastas and other undoctored foods seemed so exotic at the time, but of course are widely available now. I remember going to a fundraiser dinner where my place card read: "Alice Christensen: whole-wheat noodles"!

I was deep into Yoga practice by then, and was able to teach my son relaxation and breathing techniques in addition to improving his diet. Slowly and steadily my child grew strong on this program. I will always be grateful to Adelle for her help in our lives.

Sometimes a drastic change in diet makes people uncomfortable, but I found that as long as the basic diet was followed at home, a few deviations while away from home were not damaging. I never became one of those awful bores who constantly screamed "Don't eat that!" My son also learned to pick and choose what would be the best for him. I was careful to see that there was no deprivation. The only thing he never got was blue popsicles; I never could find anything naturally blue with which to make them! He never missed blue popsicles, though, and grew into a handsome, strong, 6'8" man with a wonderful life.

— Alice Christensen

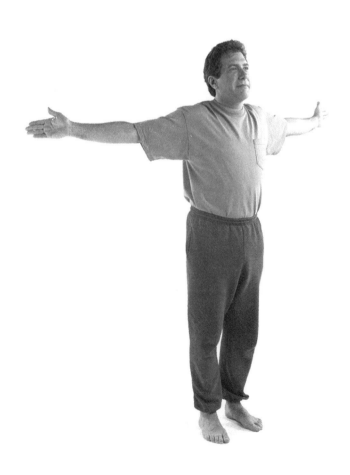

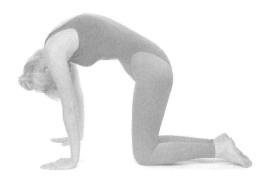

When we think of addiction, we usually think of physical dependence on alcohol, nicotine, or drugs like marijuana or heroin. People can also become addicted to caffeine, to sleeping aids, and even sugar, or to habits and behaviors that seem to bring relief from life's difficulties by avoiding change. Some examples of addictive behaviors include certain types of relationships, sex, gambling, workaholism, shopping, and so on. What people become addicted to is the experience that the substance or behavior gives them — it may make them feel stronger, more in control, more self-confident, happier, and less anxious, empty, or fearful. But the experience does not last. Addiction then becomes a way of coping with life.

Physical dependence on a substance such as nicotine, alcohol, or drugs happens when the substance begins to replace the natural chemical processes of the body and brain that determine mood and function. As the body becomes more dependent on the substance to feel normal or simply to function on a daily basis, the need for the substance increases, and if the substance is not available, the body experiences symptoms of withdrawal.

Some people seem to be more predisposed to physical and/or psychological addiction than others, although no one knows for certain why this is; some researchers have hinted at the possibility of a genetic component, and others theorize that environment and social factors play a part. Whatever the causes, addiction is a serious problem that brings with it severe depletion of the body's resources and disruption of the natural chemical balance of the body and brain.

Often an addictive substance begins to take the place of food, so the body may become quite malnourished and more susceptible to disease. Addictive substances are also used as a way of coping with stress, reducing the person's ability to deal effectively with the tasks of daily life. Because of the multiple physical and psychological components of addiction, effective treatment focuses on both the body and the mind, helping the addicted person to regain health and strength and teaching new coping skills.

• *H*ow Yoga Can Help •

Many people in recovery are quite unhealthy. A body in recovery needs care and attention through exercise, relaxation, stress-coping skills, and a balanced, healthy diet.

Any kind of addiction can be helped by the discipline and health of regular Yoga practice. Yoga helps you find relief inside yourself so you don't have to depend on an external solution. Yoga will teach you techniques that you can use throughout the day to reinforce healthy habits. Most importantly, Yoga will prevent your body from going into shock with the pain of withdrawal. As you slowly build your courage and strength by relying on your inner being, you will realize that you are on your way to recognizing the strength and power to change that is already a part of you. When you use Yoga techniques to help yourself heal, you are strengthening yourself from within. Addiction does not destroy your strength; it makes you forget about it. Yoga helps you remember that your strength resides within you, and that you can use it to grow healthy again.

Yoga frees you from addiction by giving the body and mind something else to take the place of the addictive substance — something as pleasant and stress-relieving in its way as the addictive substance you once used for relief. One of the best things you can do is the "I Love You" meditation technique (see Chapter 1). Practice this every day to improve your self-confidence and heal your self-esteem.

Yoga exercises put pressure on your glands and organs, causing a chemical change in your body that includes a very pleasurable secretion to seep into your system — the endorphins, the brain chemicals that cause feelings of well-being. In a completely individualistic way, according to your own particular body system, Yoga techniques start to balance the glandular activity. Yoga exercise also flushes the drug toxins out of your body. You will notice yourself feeling better very quickly. This is one reason why, when people practice Yoga for a while, they very seldom give it up. The feeling of well-being is delicious and remains in the forefront even through the normal upsets of daily life. It helps you to resist inevitable cravings.

Because of its subtle quality, smoking is one of the hardest addictions to give up. The urge to reach for a cigarette when you feel under stress is very strong. The Complete Breath technique is your best weapon against this urge. Simply start breathing deeply, and focus on the sound of the breath without thinking of anything else for a minute or two. The Complete Breath will relax you, take your mind temporarily off whatever is causing the stress reaction, and give you time to recover. You can do this breathing technique anywhere, anytime, and no one has to know

you're doing it. A good diet is very important in quitting smoking, especially vitamin C; many people have been helped by taking a low-dose supplement every two hours throughout the day.

Because Yoga acts as a natural stimulant by increasing your energy level, you may find yourself cutting down on your addictive consumption or behavior even without making a conscious decision to do so. As a general rule, you'll find that as you become stronger and healthier, your body will naturally tend to reject things that will harm it. Many students have told me how they thought they could never give up their five cups of coffee a day, yet one day they realized that they had cut down to two, or one, or even none without even noticing.

If you have trouble falling asleep, instead of reaching for sleeping pills, practice the Complete Breath and the relaxation and meditation procedures lying in bed. Many people have found this extremely helpful for getting back into a normal cycle of adequate rest at night. If you are suffering from "workaholism," an inability to fall asleep may simply mean that you are unable to stop thinking about work; Yoga practice can teach you to stop working when you wish to. Another useful suggestion is simply to get up, go about your normal activities, and schedule a nap during the day.

Difficulty concentrating or remembering is a common result of the unbalanced body chemistry caused by the use of addictive substances. You may also lack stamina and the ability to be flexible in difficult situations. In my experience, Yoga breathing and meditation are the best tools for reconnecting with the important qualities of concentration, memory, and adaptability. Make a commitment to practicing every day — even if it's just for a few minutes — and you will start to notice results immediately. Breathing exercises are particularly helpful. In my experience with students, alcohol problems are the most quickly affected. I have had many students present themselves to me as alcoholics who, after as little as two to three weeks of regular practice, had no further need for alcohol.

• Special Concerns •

If you are in a painful withdrawal stage, see your physician right away. Don't try to brave it out alone. Ask for help during this difficult time. Sometimes the temporary use of medication can relieve symptoms enough so that you can begin the task of rebuilding your health. If you combine this therapy with regular practice of Yoga exercises, meditation, and breathing, you will experience a great relief that hopefully will allow you to function happily without the addictive substance and, soon, without the medication as well.

• Things You Can Do Throughout the Day •

The Complete Breath is your best tool to counteract harmful stress reactions. Use it whenever you feel anxious, depressed, fearful, lonely, or bored.

Do stretching exercises several times a day to stay in touch with your body: try the Full Bend and Variation, the Standing Reach and Standing Twist, and the Lazy Stretch (see Chapter 1).

• Dietary Suggestions •

You should be eating a balanced "anti-stress" diet: rich in low-fat protein (such as low-fat dairy foods, legumes, and whole grains), fresh fruits and vegetables, and complex carbohydrates. Avoid sugary, high-fat, or artificial foods. Avoid chemicals such as artificial flavors and colors, overly processed foods, and caffeinated beverages. Learn to read labels and understand what you are putting into your body. If you can, eat several small meals throughout the day rather than three big ones, and never skip a meal. Supplement your diet with multivitamins including extra B vitamins, vitamin C, and beta-carotene. Some people have been helped by taking low doses of vitamin C every two hours throughout the day.

My teacher Rama once advised students suffering from addiction to chew on whole cloves throughout the day. I have no idea why this therapy worked, but it did.

When you are cutting down on caffeine or other stimulants, be sure you are getting more than enough protein throughout the day; this will help prevent withdrawal headaches. For the first week or so, it is helpful to count protein grams in everything you eat until you learn which foods are the best sources of protein and how much to eat every day.

Drink plenty of water throughout the day to help flush out poisons left from the addictive substance.

• Daily Routine for Recovery from Addiction •

Start with the basic routine described in Chapter 1, then incorporate the special exercises in this chapter. These exercises have been chosen because they improve circulation in order to flush toxins out of the body, increase willpower and concentration, stimulate the endocrine system, balance metabolism, and stretch and relax major muscle groups.

If you don't have time to do a full routine, do at least three warmup exercises and three of the exercises described below, and always do the complete relaxation procedure and at least a few minutes of meditation. Best results will be obtained if you practice a little every day without fail. Never do these exercises under the influence of drugs or alcohol.

Here is the full sequence of techniques (including the basic routine):

Complete Breath, p. 26
Warmups, pp. 16-20
Archer Pose, p. 35
T Pose, p. 36
Standing Sun Pose, p. 21
Stretching Dog, p. 36
Arm and Leg Balance, p. 37
Cat Breath, p. 37
Camel Pose, p. 38
Baby Pose, p. 24
Seated Sun Pose, p. 22
Tortoise Stretch, p. 23
Knee Squeeze, p. 38
Swan Dive, p. 39
Cobra Pose, p. 39
Relaxation and Meditation, pp. 26-27

Archer Pose. *Increases mental poise and one-pointedness; helps heal addiction.* The ideal position for your feet in this pose is pointed straight ahead, one directly in front of the other. Until you master the exercise, you may keep your feet slightly apart for balance. Start with the left foot forward and the right back. Extend your right arm straight ahead and position the hand as if you were holding a bow, with the thumb pointed up. Place your left hand on your head with fingers curled to hold the string of the bow (**A**). Breathe in, looking forward at your right thumb, then slowly and carefully breathe out and turn toward the right, keeping your right arm outstretched and following your thumb with your gaze. Twist back as far as you can (**B**), hold your breath out for a count of three, then inhale as you twist slowly back to face front. Relax your arms and switch positions (left hand outstretched, right hand on your head) but keep your feet in the same position. Stare at the thumb of your outstretched hand. Breathe in, then slowly and carefully twist back — to the left this time (**C**). Hold for a count of three, then breathe in and return to the front. Relax your arms. Repeat both movements with the right foot forward. [one sequence on each side]

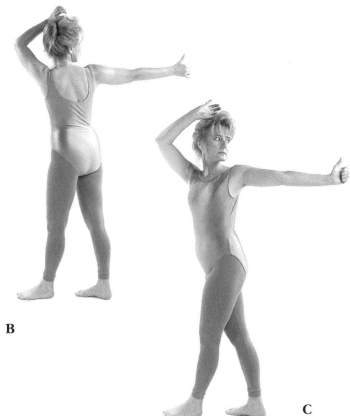

B

C

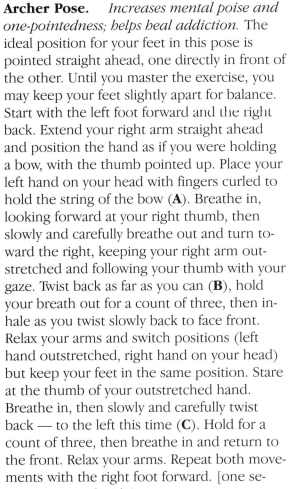

A

What to do When You Experience a Craving

When you start to feel that nothing will do but that you have to have a cigarette, a drink, or some other substance right away, try this short routine to distract you, to substitute other pleasurable feelings for the substance, and to relax your body and mind. Start by having a hot, noncaffeinated drink. Then, do:

5 Complete Breaths, focusing only on the sound of the breath.

3 Standing Sun Poses, imagining the health and energy of the sun coursing through your body and brain.

3 Archer Poses, imagining yourself taking aim against your addiction and blasting it to pieces with a flaming arrow.

Complete relaxation, lying down or seated in a chair, with no thought except the feeling of limpness as each muscle relaxes.

The "I Love You" meditation technique. (Carry our audiotape around with you if you can.)

T Pose.   *Strengthens legs and back; improves vigor; tones abdominal organs; increases concentration, memory, and mental poise.* Start by holding on to a sturdy chair or counter for support until you get more confident. Stand about three feet away from the support and lean forward. Balance on your left leg and raise your right leg in back parallel to the floor or as high as you can (**A**). It's important not to hold your breath in this exercise; let your breath relax; it will be faster due to the extra exertion required by this pose. Staring at one spot on the floor, see if you can loosen your grip on the chair. If you can, raise your arms straight in front of you and place your palms together (**B**). At first, keep your neck straight and look at a spot on the floor for balance. Later, you can try looking ahead over your two thumbs. When you are in position, hold for a count of three, then breathe out and relax. [3 times each side]

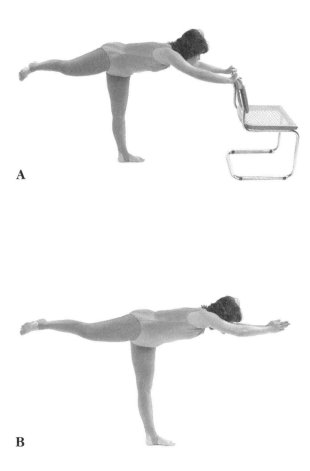

A

B

Stretching Dog.   *Limbers lower back and hips; stretches back of legs; increases circulation to head; strengthens heart.* Sit on your heels, toes tucked under and hands on the floor a few inches in front of your knees. Breathe in and arch your back, looking up (**C**). Hold for a count of three. Breathe out and straighten your legs, pushing your body into a V position (**D**). Tuck your chin and hold for a count of three. [3 repetitions]

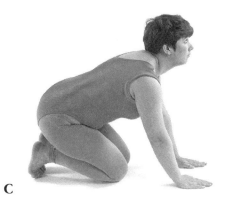

C

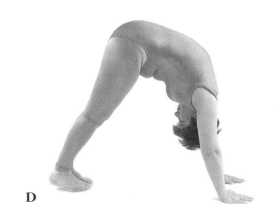

D

Arm & Leg Balance.   *Strengthens muscles of the lower and midback, strengthens legs and hips; improves concentration.* On hands and knees, breathe out completely. Then breathe in and raise your left arm and right leg parallel to the floor (**A**). Look straight ahead at your outstretched arm, or, if your balance is shaky, stare at one spot on the floor. Hold for a count of three. Breathe out and lower. Repeat with the right arm and left leg. [3 each side, alternating opposites]

If you feel very steady, you can vary this exercise by lifting the arm and leg on the same side of the body instead (**B**). [3 repetitions, each side]

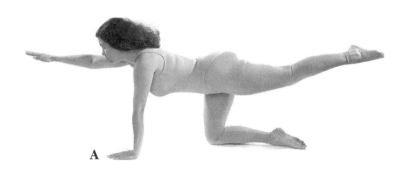

A

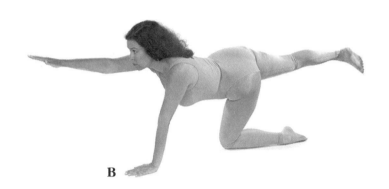

B

Cat Breath.   *Limbers lower and midback; tightens stomach muscles; improves breathing. Start on hands and knees.* Breathe in, arch your back, and look up (**C**), so you feel the stretch all along your spine from tailbone to neck. Hold for a count of three. Then breathe out, round your back, and pull up on your stomach to increase the forward stretch (**D**). Tuck your chin and hold for a count of three. [3 repetitions]

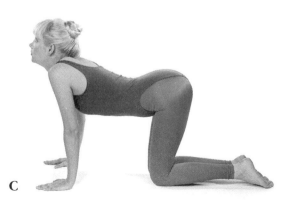

C

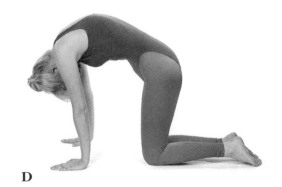

D

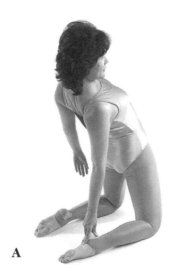

A

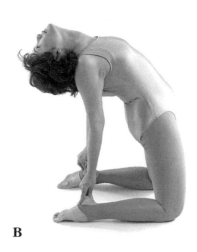

B

Camel. *Limbers entire spine; improves circulation and respiration; stretches and strengthens thighs and knees; improves functioning of thyroid; strengthens heart.* Kneel with legs slightly (**A**) separated. The first two movements in this exercise help to prepare the spine for an intense stretch: Carefully bend back and grasp your left heel with your left hand. Push your hips forward slightly. Repeat on the right side. Now bend backward and grasp one heel with each hand.

Push your hips forward as far as possible and let your head relax back (do not let your head fall back (**B**) if you have neck problems). Hold for a count of three, breathing normally. Release and rest briefly in the Baby Pose. As you get stronger, you can extend the length of the hold. [3 repetitions]

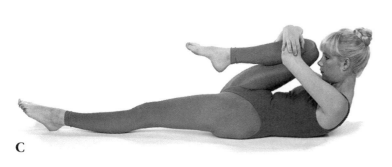

C

Knee Squeeze. *Improves digestion; limbers and relaxes lower back and hips; improves circulation in pelvic region; removes poisons from the body.* Lie on your back with arms over your head on the floor. Breathe out completely. Keeping your right knee straight, breathe in, bend your left knee, and lift your head, wrapping your arms around the knee. Hold your breath in and squeeze your knee to your chest (**C**). Hold for a count of three, then release, breathe out, and lower the leg and arms back to the starting position. [3 times each side, alternating]

After 3 repetitions on each side, do the same exercise lifting both legs at once (**D**). [3 repetitions]

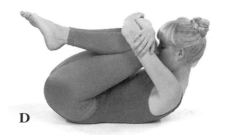

D

Swan Dive. *Strengthens back, leg, and shoulder muscles — especially helpful for lower back; massages internal organs; improves circulation to the spine and brain.* Lie on your stomach with your legs together, your arms stretched out to the sides, and your forehead on the floor. Breathe out. Breathe in as you lift arms, legs, and head, looking up through your forehead (**A**). Hold for a count of three. Breathe out and relax back to the starting position. [3 repetitions]

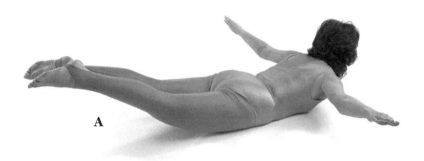

A

Cobra Pose. *Improves functioning of digestive, respiratory, and reproductive systems; limbers and strengthens entire spine; strengthens eyesight; equalizes two sides of body; improves complexion.* Lie on your stomach with legs together (those with occasional lower back trouble should separate the legs at first). Place your forehead on the floor and your palms underneath your shoulders close to your body so your elbows point up, not out to the sides (**B**). Breathe out completely, then start to breathe in as you curl first your head and eyes back as far as they will go, then your chest, and then your stomach (**C**). Keep your hipbones on the floor — this is not a push-up — and your arms slightly bent (unless you are extremely limber). Use your back muscles more than your arms. Hold for a count of three with your breath in and eyes looking up through

your forehead. Do not blink. Then start to breathe out and curl forward slowly, in reverse: your stomach curls down first, then your chest, and finally your head and eyes. Your eyes are the first part of your body to curl up and the last to curl down. [3 repetitions]

Caution: This is a very powerful exercise and should not be done if you have had recent surgery or by women during the menstrual period, as it increases blood flow.

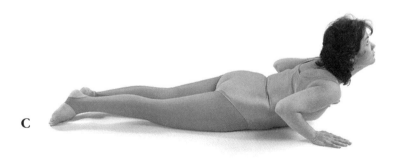

C

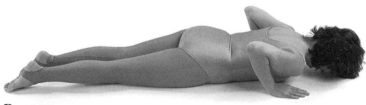

B

Yoga practice is most effective if done every day, even if you have time for only a few techniques. Many people believe that if they don't have time to practice the entire routine, it isn't worth doing anything at all. This is not true. Yoga works on a cumulative basis, so a daily remembrance of even a few techniques adds to the benefits of Yoga over time.

The best way to instill a regular Yoga routine is to do it at the same time every day, until it becomes a habit, just like combing your hair. Even better, if you can, split your Yoga practice into segments that you do twice a day — for instance, breathing and meditation in the morning and exercises when you get home from work. Besides giving you more energy and strength and happiness to improve your day, you'll get in the habit of doing healthy things every day — and enjoying them as well. The more you remember to breathe, to exercise, and to meditate regularly, the better you'll feel. There's nothing wrong with becoming addicted to this type of feeling!

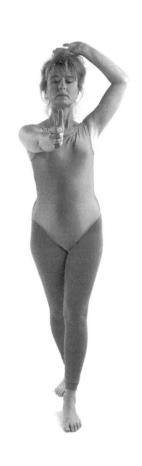

There is a line in *The Bhagavad Gita* (an ancient text about Yoga) that says that Yoga is meant for the person who doesn't eat too much or too little, who doesn't sleep too much or too little, who is moderate in all things. There is a great value in learning that you don't have to be perfect; that you can allow yourself occasional indulgence — as long as what you are indulging in is not destructive. Many people, especially those in recovery who find that they must completely abstain from alcohol or other addictive substances in order to remain healthy, translate that all-or-nothing approach into all other areas of their lives. If you are trying to reduce your intake of "junk food," for instance, you may think that you must never, ever have another cookie or doughnut or potato chip. An attitude like this is a type of violence to yourself, because it relies on guilt and punishment rather than conscious choice. It is true that some personalities are more prone to excess than others and you may not be able to "eat just one" at first. But with time, and with daily practice of Yoga, you will build willpower and concentration, and become more trusting of your own judgment in making healthy choices, bringing balance and enjoyment into your life.

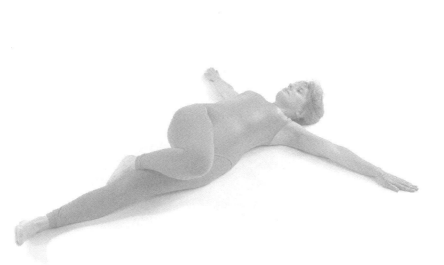

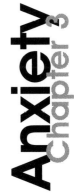

*E*veryone suffers from mild anxiety from time to time, but chronic anxiety takes a tremendous toll on the body, draining energy resources and keeping the body in a constant state of stress. Anxiety is related to fear — but an important difference is that fear is usually taken to be a normal response to a real danger, while anxiety is a feeling in which the threat is not readily apparent, yet the person experiences greater-than-expected worry, uncertainty, and fear. Whether the fear is real or imagined, however, your body and mind experience it the same way.

A "panic attack" occurs when the fear becomes so intense that you become paralyzed. About 15 million Americans say they have experienced a panic attack at least once in their lives. Usually, a panic attack lasts only a few seconds, but the anxiety, dread, embarrassment, and despair that accompany it can last for several minutes, hours, or even days. Just the fear of having such an attack can cause an anxiety reaction. Even when you take steps to avoid situations that may be anxiety producing, you can increase the significance of that situation until it becomes impossible for you to think about it without becoming anxious and debilitated. You become a prisoner of your own fears.

Anxiety is generally considered undesirable, but there are situations in which people consciously seek out anxious feelings — such as those who practice risky careers or sports, for instance, or performers — because the extra adrenaline sharpens concentration and performance.

Anxiety produces physical symptoms such as paleness, sweating, dilation of pupils, and rapid heartbeat. The effects of anxiety are magnified when the body is not exercised: tension in the muscles builds, breathing remains constricted most of the time, and the mind has no rest from the whirling thoughts and feelings that feed the anxiety. If the anxiety or fear continues for a long time, you become fatigued and depressed; you may lose your appetite, your ability to concentrate, and your ability to sleep restfully.

Telling yourself to "just get over it" is not an effective approach. Fear deserves respect, just as you respect your other feelings. Respect both the "rational" fears and the "irrational" ones. Both are real to you in some way, and both can cause debilitating physical reactions. If you get panic attacks often, your self-esteem may plummet as you think that there must be something wrong with you. Often people turn to alcohol or drugs out of desperation for something to calm their fears; fear is one of the major causes of addiction and can also lead to other self-destructive behaviors.

• *H*ow Yoga Can Help •

One reason anxiety attacks are so painful is because they make you feel like a victim. Yoga helps you to access an inner strength that enables you to face the sometimes overwhelming fears, frustrations, and challenges of everyday life. Yoga reduces stress in the body, breath, and mind by building coping skills with a small daily routine of exercise, breathing, and meditation.

A few Yoga exercises practiced daily (especially if they are done just prior to meditation) help to regulate the breath and relax the body by gently releasing tension from the large muscle groups, flushing all parts of the body and brain with fresh blood, oxygen, and other nutrients, and increasing feelings of well-being. "Whole body" exercises such as the Sun Poses are particularly helpful because they encourage you to breathe deeply and rhythmically. Yoga exercises balance the glandular changes of the body that occur in response to stress and anxiety. Many exercises can be adapted so you can do them even in an office chair for help throughout the day.

The Complete Breath technique (see p. 26) is a must for anyone who often feels "stressed out." Once learned, the Complete Breath can be used anywhere, anytime, to reduce the severity of a panic attack, to calm the mind, or to cope with a difficult situation. Learning to concentrate simply on the sound of the breath as you inhale and exhale evenly and smoothly will help you gently but effectively switch your attention from feelings of anxiety to feelings of relaxation.

Daily practice of complete relaxation and meditation is also essential — even a few minutes of meditation during your work day can make a difference. This daily training in focusing the mind on stillness will teach you how to consciously quiet your mind whenever you feel overwhelmed. Meditation puts you in touch with your inner resources; this means less dependence on medications, greater self-awareness, and a fuller, happier, less anxious life.

When you feel overwhelmed by anxiety, negative thoughts crowd out the positive ones. Many experts agree that reversing that process by consciously making positive statements to yourself can change how you feel about yourself. Yoga gives you different ways of giving your body and mind positive statements. Yoga exercises, for instance, are positive messages to the body. They protect against the "cliffhanger" feeling of anxiety by providing a constant balance and support from within the body with a strong and resilient nervous system. Yoga meditation teaches the mind to listen to the healing messages of silence.

Special Concerns

If your anxiety is so severe that it paralyzes you, preventing you from doing the normal tasks of life, seek professional counseling as soon as possible. Your Yoga routine will support your progress toward better health as you work with a counselor to reduce your fears.

Things You Can Do Throughout the Day

When you find yourself obsessing about the past or future, use exercise, breathing, or meditation to help you stay in the present. The best techniques are the Complete Breath, the Standing Sun Pose, and meditation.

You can use fantasy to help you replace negative thoughts with positive ones. When you catch yourself having frequent anxious thoughts about some future event, sit in a quiet room for a few minutes, close your eyes, and imagine yourself succeeding. Remember a situation in which you surprised yourself by doing something you didn't think you could. Post a note reminding yourself of this situation on your refrigerator or some other place where you will see it several times a day.

Learn to recognize your body's signals that anxiety is beginning to build: increased heart rate, tense muscles, whirling or repetitive thoughts, and so on. As soon as you identify a panic-triggering thought or physical sensation, immediately begin the Complete Breath and you may be able to stop the sequence of events that leads to a panic attack.

Replace your morning coffee break with a Yoga break. In 15 minutes, you can do a few exercises, a few Complete Breaths, and a few minutes of meditation.

Dietary Suggestions

Some researchers have found a link between sensitivity to substances called lactates and increased anxiety. Elevated levels of lactates can be caused by alcohol, caffeine, sugar, deficiency of B vitamins and calcium or magnesium, and food allergies. People who are under constant stress are very likely to be deficient in many nutrients because the body is continually responding with the "fight or flight" syndrome, using up the body's resources quickly in order to be ready for action. If you suffer from repeated anxiety attacks, examine your diet closely. Eat a balanced, healthy diet rich in protein, B vitamins, and calcium; if you can, eat several small nutritious meals throughout the day rather than two or three large ones. Whole grains, fresh vegetables and fruits, and foods high in the B vitamins are especially nutritious. Consider supplementing your diet with extra B-complex vitamins, calcium, and magnesium in small doses throughout the day.

• Daily Routine for Anxiety •

Start with the basic routine described in Chapter 1, then incorporate the special exercises in this chapter. These exercises have been chosen because they improve circulation, help you identify and relax tension in major muscle groups, increase concentration on the present moment to release fear associated with past or future thoughts, improve respiration through compression and whole-body exercises, and help you practice general stress-coping skills that reduce the time needed for recovery.

If you don't have time to do a full routine, do at least three warmup exercises and three of the exercises described below, and always do at least a few minutes of meditation. Best results will be obtained if you practice every day. Many of the exercises below can be done in chairs.

Here is a list of the full sequence of techniques (including the basic routine):

Dancer Pose. *Strengthens the lower back; limbers and strengthens the hips and thighs; improves mental poise; improves posture, balance, and concentration; strengthens ankles; relieves upper back tension.* Throughout the exercise, steady yourself by fixing your gaze on one spot on the wall in front of you. From a standing rest position, bend your right knee and grasp your right foot in back with your left hand (**A**). Check to be sure your stomach muscles are relaxed and your breathing steady. Slowly move into the completed Dancer Pose by raising your right arm straight up toward the ceiling so it is next to your ear and pulling your right leg up and back as far as possible without strain (**B**). Don't lean forward, and keep your supporting leg straight. Relax your stomach, breathe normally, and keep your gaze fixed on one spot. Hold for a count of three, then carefully return to the beginning position. [3 times each side]

Dancer Pose Extension. *Try this extension after you have become proficient in the Dancer Pose.* From the Dancer position after your three-count hold as described above, maintain your gaze and, still breathing normally, slowly lower your body into the extended position (**C**). In addition to the benefits of the Dancer Pose, this variation stretches the back of the legs and increases strength and stamina. Keep your right leg as far up and back as possible. Your right arm extends straight ahead. Your left (supporting) leg remains straight. Hold for a count of three. Stare at one spot for balance. Don't strain. Come back to a standing rest position.

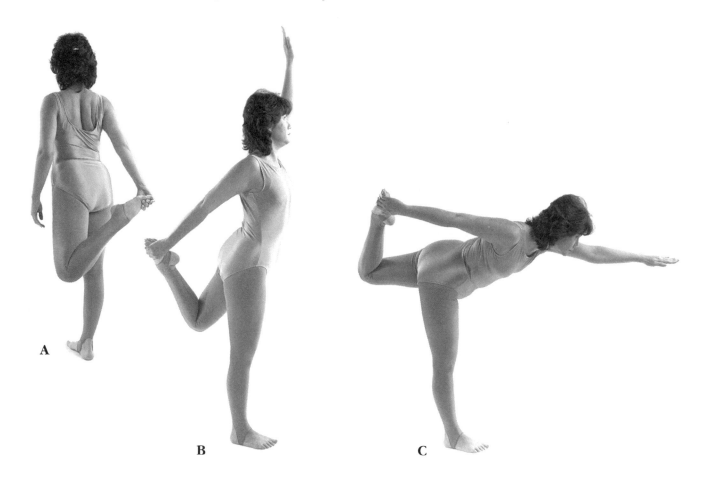

A

B

C

Twisting Triangle. *Increases flexibility and circulation in hips and lower back; strengthens hip joints and upper back; helps relieve depression.* Separate your feet as wide as you can comfortably (without losing your balance) and point your toes forward. Breathe in and raise your arms to the sides, parallel to the floor (**A**). Breathe out as you bend toward the left leg, grasp the outside of your left ankle (or calf) with your right hand, then turn your head so you are looking at your left hand, which should be pointed straight up toward the ceiling, fingers curled and thumb toward you (**B**). Stare at your thumb. You can pull slightly with your right hand to increase the stretch. Keep both knees straight. Hold for a count of three, then breathe in and come back to your starting position, arms outstretched. [3 times each side, alternating]

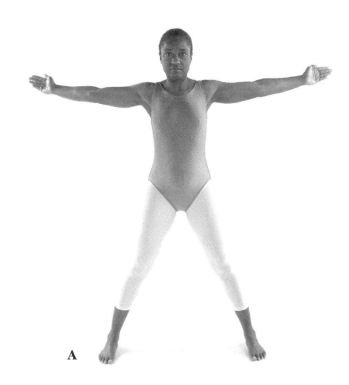

A

B

A Teacher's Experience

Teaching is one of the most stressful professions due to the high number of interpersonal interactions. The Complete Breath, practiced every day, was the most vivid sign of the benefits of Yoga for me as a teacher. I was a beginning teacher and used to become quite tense in my abdominal region every day whenever some disruption occurred. After practicing about one or two months I noticed that my abdomen would automatically relax each time it tightened up, because of the movements I learned in doing the Complete Breath. I also found my creative energy depleted very quickly because of the constant demand to keep order in a large classroom. My daily practice of meditation became very important to me over time because it replenished that well of creativity.

— A. C., elementary school
teacher in Cleveland, Ohio

Arm & Leg Balance. *Strengthens muscles of the lower and midback, strengthens legs and hips; improves concentration.* On hands and knees, breathe out completely. Then breathe in and raise your left arm and right leg parallel to the floor (**A**). Look straight ahead at your outstretched arm, or, if your balance is shaky, stare at one spot on the floor. Hold for a count of three. Breathe out and lower. Repeat with the right arm and left leg. [3 each side, alternating opposites] If you feel very steady, you can vary this exercise by lifting the arm and leg on the same side of the body instead (**B**). [3 repetitions, each side]

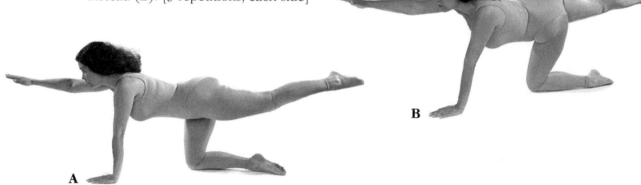

B

A

Bow Variation. *Strengthens vertebrae, back and shoulder muscles, and hips and thighs; improves balance and memory.* Start on hands and knees, with hands supporting you about shoulder width apart. Reach back with your right hand and grasp your left foot. Breathe in as you lift the foot up away from your body, arching your back a little (**C**). Hold for a count of three. Breathe out and relax. [3 times each side, alternating]

C

Spine Twist. *Improves digestion; limbers and tones entire spine; strengthens and limbers rib cage; relieves chronic constipation; helps relieve bladder, urinary tract, and prostate problems; strengthens heart.* Bend both knees. Rest your right leg on the floor, and lift your left leg over the right knee; the left foot should be flat (**A**). Sit up very straight, reach your right arm across your left knee, push the knee as far right as it will go, and grasp your left ankle; this locks the lower back into position (**B**). (Alternatively, if you are unable to reach your left ankle, grasp your right knee instead. You can also simply hook your right arm over your left knee and straighten the leg, as in (**D**). Now place your left arm behind you, straighten it and point the fingers in toward the base of your spine. Look forward, breathe in, then breathe out and twist toward the left as far as possible. Look far to the left with your eyes and stare at one spot (**C**). Hold for a count of three, breathing gently. As you get stronger, you can increase the holding time. Then release and slowly come forward. [3 times to each side]

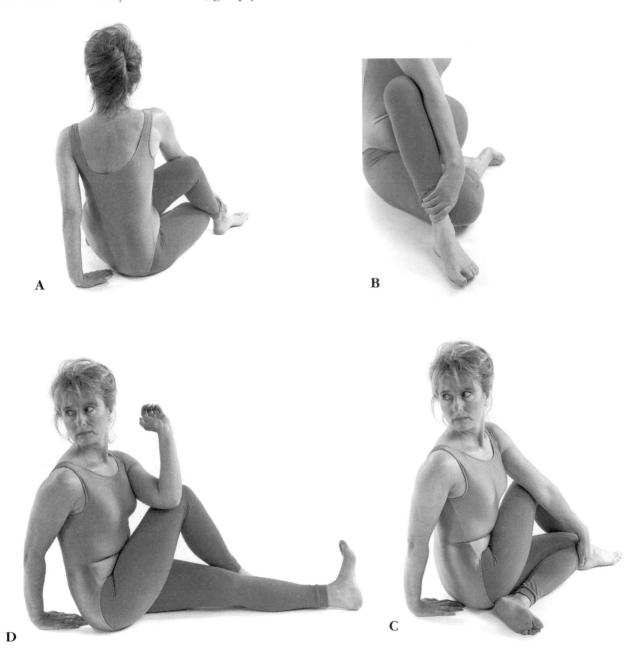

A

B

D

C

Eye Palming. *Relaxes tension in face and eyes.* To relieve tension around your eyes at any time of day, place your palms gently over your closed eyes and hold for 10 to 30 seconds (**A**).

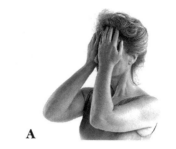

A

Knee Squeeze. *Improves digestion; limbers and relaxes lower back and hips; improves circulation in pelvic region; removes poisons from the body.* Lie on your back with arms over your head on the floor. Breathe out completely. Keeping your right knee straight, breathe in, bend your left knee, and lift your head, wrapping your arms around the knee (**B**). Hold your breath in and squeeze your knee to your chest. Hold for a count of three, then release, breathe out, and lower the leg and arms back to the starting position. [3 times each side, alternating]

After 3 repetitions on each side, do the same exercise lifting both legs at once (**C**). [3 repetitions]

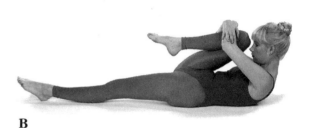

B

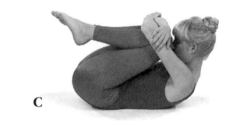

C

Lower Back Stretch. *Improves functioning of internal organ; improves circulation; strengthens and limbers the shoulders, back, and hip joints; helps to trim the waistline.* If you have a spinal disk problem, be very careful with this exercise. Lie on your back with your legs together and arms stretched out to the sides, palms down. Breathe out, then breathe in as you lift your left leg and hook your left toe under your right knee. Breathe out as you bend your left leg to the right over your right leg toward the floor as far as possible without straining (**D**). Keep your shoulders and arms on the floor and keep your right leg straight. Hold the position and your breath for a count of three. Breathe in as you roll back, lift your left knee up, and straighten your leg toward the ceiling. Breathe out as you return the leg to the floor. [3 times each side, alternating]

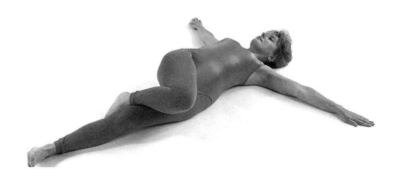

D

Boat Pose. *Strengthens back muscles, improves digestion and functioning of all internal organs.* Lie on your stomach, forehead to the floor and arms stretched out in front. Breathe out, then breathe in and lift your arms, legs, and head (**A**). Look up. Hold your breath and the position for a count of three, then breathe out and lower to your starting position. [3 repetitions]

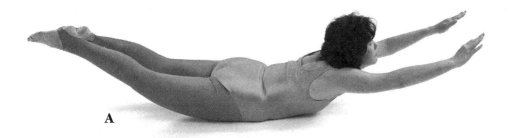

A

Yoga Throughout the Day

You will greatly increase the effects of Yoga practice if you remember to apply the techniques not just for 20 or 30 minutes once a day, but whenever you need them throughout the day. If you work at a desk or computer for long hours, for example, get in the habit of doing a few exercises every hour or so to keep muscles from becoming tight. The Shoulder Roll (p. 16), Neck Stretch (p. 17), Seated Knee Squeeze (p. 107), and Seated Twist (p. 107) are some examples of exercises that can be done in a chair.

Whenever you find yourself with time on your hands, such as while waiting in a doctor's office, waiting for a traffic light to change, and so on, instead of letting feelings of impatience and tension build, remember to practice your Complete Breath. You'll strengthen your respiratory system while reducing the tight stomach muscles that can contribute to harmful stress reactions.

Use balance poses, such as the Tree Pose (p. 82) and T Pose (p. 36), to quiet racing thoughts. These exercises steady your nervous system from the inside out. If you don't have a private place to exercise when you feel stressed, just sit quietly for a moment and try to recall the feeling of quietness and calmness that you experience when you meditate. Simply remembering that feeling will bring back its relaxing qualities.

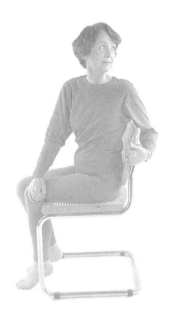

Arthritis
Chapter 4

Most people use the term "arthritis" to mean any painful condition of the joints, bones, or muscles, including bursitis, rheumatism, gout, and tendinitis, among many others. Diseases such as fibromyalgia or severe allergies also can cause arthritislike symptoms. Approximately 37 million people in this country experience some form of the hundred or so diseases we call arthritis.

The term "arthritis" means inflammation of the joints. Rheumatoid arthritis is a more severe form of inflammation that can affect other organs and tissues in the body besides the joints. Arthritis can be caused by such varied factors as heredity, a malfunctioning immune system, the natural wear and tear of joints over time, infections, environmental reactions, injuries, and perhaps even allergic reactions to certain foods.

Arthritis affects people of all ages, though people over 50 are more likely to have osteoarthritis, which results from daily wear and tear on the joints. Osteoarthritis is the most common form of the disease; over 16 million Americans are currently diagnosed with it. Rheumatoid arthritis commonly afflicts younger people, primarily women. It is a chronic condition that can be successfully controlled but usually not cured.

Arthritis that is due to an infection may be prevented or cured with a course of antibiotics. Conditions like bursitis and tendinitis, that are usually confined to one joint, will often respond completely to a short period of rest. Even the chronic forms of arthritis,

though, can usually be kept in check with a careful program that combines exercise, good nutrition, and rest, as well as awareness and protection of the joints.

Some arthritislike conditions, such as gout, are caused by crystallization of certain blood chemicals when levels become too high. The crystals, which form in the joints, irritate the lining and cause severe inflammation. The joint becomes swollen, red, and painful. A careful program of exercise, diet, and stress management will help balance the body's chemistry and help prevent this problem from developing. Yoga exercises are designed to help balance the glandular systems of the body.

Getting enough exercise is important for those with arthritis, even though you may not feel like exercising due to pain or stiffness. Equally as important as adequate activity is getting enough rest. Especially with an inflammatory condition such as rheumatoid arthritis, you will have to learn to pace yourself. Too much inactivity, however, is just as bad for you as too much stress on the joints. When a joint becomes immobilized for too long, its functioning will become greatly diminished — sometimes permanently. Stretching exercises are particularly important. By moving your joints regularly, you keep them mobile and strengthen the surrounding muscles. Weight-bearing exercises reduce your risk of osteoporosis, or brittle bones, which is sometimes associated with arthritis. Moving your joints also distributes nutrients and waste products to and from your cartilage, the important cushioning material on the ends of bones that keeps them loose, comfortable, and mobile. The compression poses of Yoga are effective because they aid in the circulation of blood to all the extremities.

During a flare-up of arthritis, you may have to reduce your exercise program slightly. During those times, try to continue exercising a little every day. All Yoga exercises can be modified for days when you are feeling more fragile. Regular exercise is essential for maintaining good posture as well, which eases the burden on your back muscles and your spine.

If you are troubled by stiffness in the morning, try doing a few exercises while lying in bed or during a hot shower. Some have found that doing a few exercises in the evening just before bed can also reduce morning stiffness. See Appendix A for some exercises that can be done in bed.

• *H*ow Yoga Can Help •

Arthritis can be experienced as a minor nuisance, or it can be incapacitating. Most physicians agree that the stretching exercises of Yoga can be beneficial for osteoarthritis because they keep muscle tone intact and help to prevent stiffness in the joints. If you have rheumatoid arthritis, you may need to begin more slowly with an exercise program, concentrating more on the breathing and relaxation aspects.

When the pain of arthritis strikes, it has an effect of stiffening up the rest of the body, as if to protect the part that hurts. Most people respond to this by decreasing their activity level. Inactivity, however, is often the worst thing to do because it weakens the muscles and actually increases stiffness and pain. Yoga encourages you to keep moving gently while your body is healing in order to maintain muscle tone, good circulation, and joint flexibility. A regular exercise program is also extremely valuable psychologically because it increases your confidence that even though you have arthritis, you're not going to be a prisoner in a wheelchair; you can work, play, and do all your daily activities if you exercise regularly.

Yoga exercises each have a particular breathing pattern, which helps bring fresh blood and nutrients to muscle tissue as well as improving respiration and relieving physical and emotional tension. Yoga exercises improve strength, flexibility, and balance. The routine in this chapter also includes instructions in self-massage to help bring warmth and improved circulation to the joints before, during, and after exercise — or any time of the day. If you have trouble getting on the floor because of arthritis in your hips or knees, many of the exercises in this chapter can be done in chairs.

Breathing, relaxation, and meditation techniques will be an important part of your daily routine: these techniques improve respiration, relieve anxiety, and can help distract attention from pain. Breathing helps to relax both physical and emotional tension by flooding the body and brain with oxygen. In Yoga you learn breathing and relaxation techniques you can use anywhere, anytime to relieve stress and tension. A regular daily practice of meditation — simply a quieting of thoughts and memories for a few minutes at a time — gives the body time to relax and heal. Meditation is a complete rest for body and mind and will help counteract feelings of depression, anger, and helplessness that often appear when a chronic disease strikes.

Arthritis does not have to be a disability; by practicing a few gentle exercises, breathing, and meditation every day, you can reduce pain, build your strength, and maintain your daily activities with health and renewed energy.

• *S*pecial Concerns •

Because the forms and symptoms of arthritis vary, and because sometimes arthritislike symptoms can be signs of more serious disease, never attempt to diagnose yourself. If you believe you may have arthritis, consult your physician for verification. If you try a Yoga routine, remember to start slowly, but be regular about practicing every day — even if it's just a few minutes a day sometimes. Don't do the exercises when your joints are swollen, hot, or tender; exercise when pain and stiffness are at a minimum.

Things You Can Do Throughout the Day

If you lead a sedentary lifestyle, get up every hour and move around. Do some simple stretching and bending exercises to increase blood flow to all parts of your body. Over the course of a day, do exercises that put your joints through their full range of motion. Breathe deeply through your nose and imagine the oxygen bringing healing nutrients into the muscles, joints, and bones.

At least twice a day, do the complete relaxation and meditation session. This will teach you to become more aware of how your joints and muscles feel throughout the day so you can relax tension before it can cause pain.

Dietary Suggestions

It is very important for anyone with arthritis to follow an anti-stress diet that is rich in protein, B vitamins, calcium, and other essential nutrients. See Adelle Davis's book *Let's Get Well* for a very effective program to counteract the ravages of arthritis. Avoid caffeine, alcohol, and excess sugar. Eat a diet low in saturated fats and try to maintain your ideal weight. Some sufferers experience flare-ups in response to certain foods such as milk, meat, or some vegetables. If you think diet may be a factor in your arthritis, consult a reputable nutritionist.

Sometimes allergy attacks mimic arthritic symptoms. An allergy can appear at any time in life. Consult an allergist to see if this might be a factor in your arthritis.

Daily Routine for Arthritis

Start with the basic routine described in Chapter 1, then incorporate the special exercises in this chapter. These exercises have been chosen because they improve circulation, gently stretch and relax major joints and muscles, teach self-massage, and provide range-of-motion exercises for your joints. Begin every Yoga session with a warmup routine and some breathing exercises (see Chapter 1) and end your session with meditation (also discussed in Chapter 1). If you don't have time to do a full routine, do at least three warmup exercises and three of the exercises in this chapter, and always do at least a few minutes of meditation. Best results will be obtained by practicing every day. (Many exercises can be done in a chair or even in bed. See Appendix A for suggested routines.)

Here is a list of the full sequence of techniques (including the basic routine):

Complete Breath, p. 26
Warmups, pp. 16-20
Hip Rotation, p. 53
Elbow Roll, p. 53
Standing Sun Pose, p. 21 (This exercise can also be done seated in a sturdy, straight chair with knees separated and hips pressed against the back of the chair.)
Baby Pose, p. 24 (This exercise can also be done in a chair. Sit with hips pressed against the chair back and feet flat. Lean forward over your knees and let your head and arms hang relaxed.)
Cat Breath, p. 53
Spine Twist, p. 56 (See below for a seated variation.)
Foot Flap and Ankle Rotation, p. 54
Seated Sun Pose, p. 22
Tortoise Stretch, p. 23
Massage, pp. 54-55
Easy Cobra, p. 57
Relaxation and Meditation, pp. 26-27

Hip Rotation. *Limbers lower back and hip joints, increases circulation in pelvic region, gently stretches groin muscles.* Stand with feet apart as far as you can comfortably, hands on hips with thumbs forward, so fingers support lower back (**A**). Gently rotate hips forward and back three times, and side to side three times, then in circles three times each direction. Don't strain or pull.

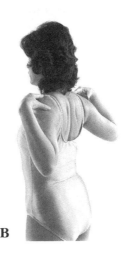

B

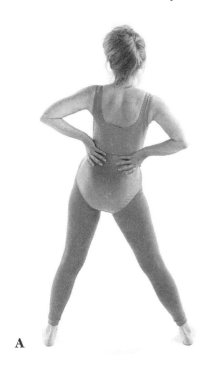

A

Elbow Roll. *Limbers shoulders and upper back; stretches chest muscles; improves breathing.* Bring the tips of your fingers to the tops of your shoulders and extend your elbows straight out horizontally (**B**). Slowly move your elbows in circles, starting with small circles and working up to larger ones. Do several circles in each direction.

Cat Breath. *Limbers lower and midback; tightens stomach muscles; improves breathing.* Start on hands and knees. Breathe in, arch your back, and look up, so you feel the stretch all along your spine from tailbone to neck (**C**). Hold for a count of three. Then breathe out, round your back, and pull up on your stomach to increase the forward stretch (**D**). Tuck your head and hold for a count of three. [3 repetitions] (For a variation that can be done in a chair, see the Frog Pose, p. 105.)

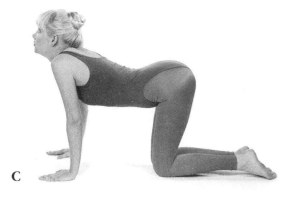

C

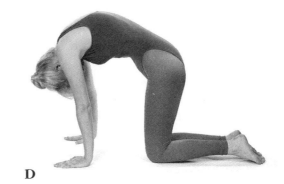

D

Foot Flap and Ankle Rotation. *Limbers and strengthens ankle and calf muscles, and improves circulation in the extremities.* Sit up straight with legs outstretched. Push your toes forward and pull them back (**A**), several times, stretching as far as possible in each direction. Now rotate each ankle in turn, three times in one direction, then three times in the other direction. This exercise can be done sitting in a chair or lying in bed.

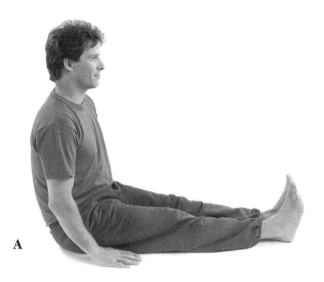

A

Massage. *Helps remove stiffness in the joints and muscles and improves circulation, making exercise easier and more pleasant, and reducing strain and injury. Helps keep you in touch with your physical body, which leads to greater self-esteem.* The point of this exercise is not to press hard with the hands and fingers but simply to increase warmth in the affected area. Use your whole hand — primarily the palm — when rubbing a joint, not just the fingers. Each joint should be massaged for at least 15 seconds. This exercise can be done throughout the day as needed.

Shoulders: Start by supporting your right elbow in your left hand. With your right hand, gently rub your left shoulder (**B**) using your whole hand — not just the fingers. Rub the entire joint for about 30 seconds. Repeat on the right side.

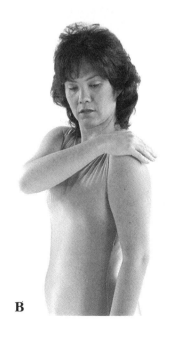

B

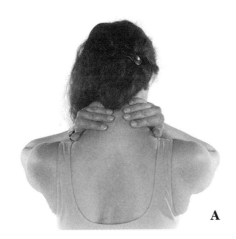

Neck: Rub the right side and back of your neck with your right hand (**A**). Use your palm. Rub for at least 30 seconds. Repeat on the left side.

Lower back: Place both hands on your lower back and rub firmly up and down all the way to the tailbone, using your palms.

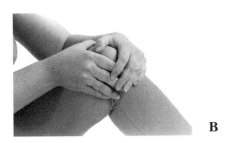

A

Knees and ankles: Massage one knee at a time. Place both hands on your knee. Rub up with one hand and down with the other hand simultaneously in a semicircular motion over the entire knee area (**B**). Use your palm. Massage ankles similarly (**C**).

B

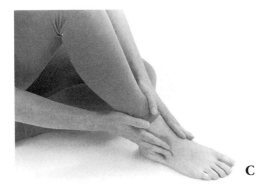

C

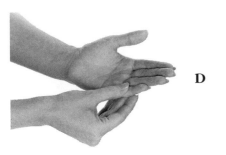

D

Hands: With your right thumb, rub your left palm and wrist, using a circular motion. Then, starting at the base of your left thumb, use your right thumb on top and right fingers underneath to rub firmly in a circular motion all over and around the joint. Move up the thumb rubbing the same way at each knuckle joint. Repeat with each of your fingers, starting from the base of each (**D**).

Finish by shaking your hands loosely.

Spine Twist. *Improves digestion; limbers and tones entire spine; strengthens and limbers rib cage; relieves chronic constipation; helps relieve bladder, urinary tract, and prostate problems; strengthens heart.* Bend both knees. Rest your right leg on the floor, and lift your left leg over the right knee; the left foot should be flat (**A**). Sit up very straight, reach your right arm across your left knee, push the knee as far right as it will go, and grasp your left ankle; this locks the lower back into position (**B**). (Alternatively, if you are unable to reach your left ankle, grasp your right knee instead. You can also simply hook your right arm over your left knee and straighten the leg, as in **C**.) Now place your left arm behind you, straighten it and point the fingers in toward the base of your spine. Look forward, breathe in, then breathe out and twist toward the left as far as possible. Look far to the left with your eyes and stare at one spot (**D**). Hold for a count of three, breathing gently, and do not blink. As you get stronger, you can increase the holding time. Then release and slowly come forward. [3 times each direction]

For the **Seated Twist** variation, sit up straight in a chair without leaning against the back. Place your right hand across your left knee and drape your left arm over the back of the chair or inside the back; the idea is to bring your left shoulder as far back as possible without strain. Now breathe in looking forward, then breathe out and twist left (toward the arm that is on the back of the chair) as far as possible without strain (**E**). Hold for a count of three, staring at one spot at eye level. Do not blink. Release. [3 repetitions each direction]

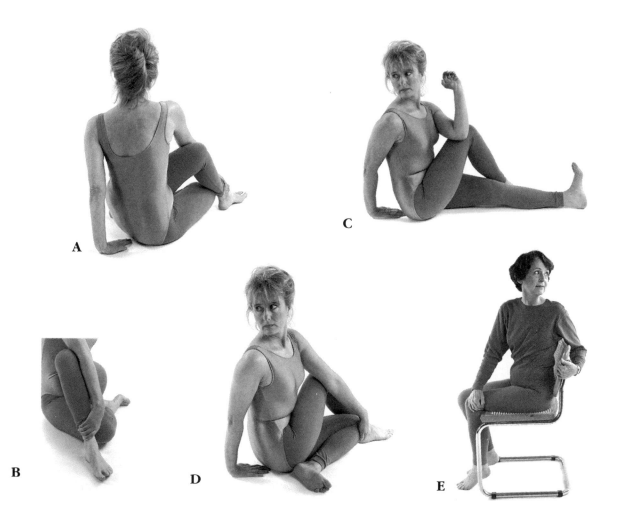

A

B

C

D

E

Easy Cobra. *Gently limbers entire spine, balances both halves of body, improves circulation, massages all internal organs; helps increase lung capacity.* Lie on your stomach resting on your forearms with hands clasped and elbows on the floor just below your shoulders, fairly close to your body. Breathe out and let your head and upper back relax forward (**A**). Now breathe in and lift your head and eyes up and back as far as possible without strain, then continue breathing in, arching your back and stretching up on your elbows, so you feel a slight stretch along your entire spinal column (**B**). Do not strain. Hold for a count of three and do not blink. Breathe out and relax your back, then your head and eyes, until your forehead comes back down to your clasped hands. Caution: this exercise should not be done if you have had recent surgery or by women during the menstrual period, as it increases blood flow. [3 repetitions] This exercise can be done in bed on a firm mattress.

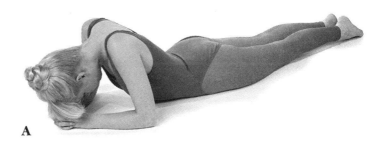

A

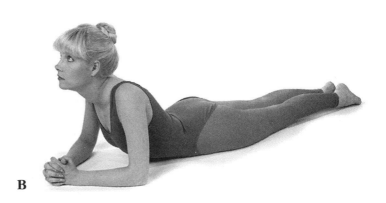

B

Asthma and Breathing Disorders
Chapter 5

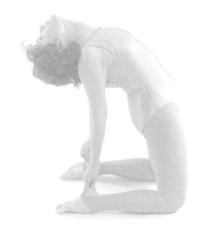

Chronic obstructive pulmonary disease (COPD) is a term that includes asthma, bronchitis, or emphysema. COPD is characterized by tightness in the chest, difficulty breathing, and often coughing and wheezing. Asthma is probably the most common of the chronic breathing disorders: between 4% and 7% of the population in the United States — approximately 10 million people — suffer from asthma.

You can develop asthma or other breathing problems simply from an irritation caused by things such as an allergy to a particular food, pollen, or medication. An underlying disease can also cause breathing disorders. Many sources believe that asthma, in particular, develops from a combination of psychological and organic causes.

Exercise is recommended for people with COPD in order to increase endurance, lessen the severity of symptoms, and reduce the number of hospital visits. Begin any exercise program very moderately. You may find it beneficial to use your inhaler before beginning to exercise. This will help you exercise longer and with less shortness of breath. Warm up and cool down thoroughly, and approach any cardiovascular or strength training with particular care. Pay attention to your breathing.

Even those who are bedridden can do an exercise routine. Many exercises can be done in bed or adapted for the bed (see Appendix A for suggestions). If the routine in this chapter is too strenuous for you, break down the exercises into smaller segments. For instance, if you can't stand up to do the Standing Sun Pose, lie on your side and practice just the arm movements, with the proper breathing pattern, with one arm at a time.

• How Yoga Can Help •

When asthma — or any chronic physical condition — strikes, it is as if you were suddenly trying to operate your car with only three wheels. Your system has been crippled. When something as strong as an asthma condition appears in your life, it does not allow you to experience your life holistically, because one system is demanding all your attention. During crisis times, you can't think about anything else, and you miss a great deal of happiness and fulfillment in your life. In order to function best, the whole being must be strong, healthy, and balanced. Yoga practice helps you to create a balanced system for body and mind.

Although COPD cannot, in most cases, be cured, the symptoms can be relieved so that attacks become less frequent and, when they do occur, can be quieted more easily. The organic causes of asthma can sometimes be helped by strengthening the body's nervous and circulatory systems. Severe allergic reactions can often be curtailed by inducing the mental quiet of meditation combined with the improved circulation of compression poses such as the Knee Squeeze.

A subtle contributor to breathing problems is the psychological impact of emotional stress. Most of us accept stress as a necessary component of our existence — and in fact, stress can be positive as well as negative. Many of us lead more highly pressured lives than we might wish for, and, although many of us are aware of the harmful effects of stress, very few of us know how to prevent or alleviate them. Your best protection against the harmful effects of stress is daily practice of a Yoga routine that includes compression exercises, regulated breathing techniques, and a period of meditation. In time, the techniques will become automatic, especially in times of stress.

Yoga teaches you to take time out for yourself to rest. You need time to daydream; to do nothing. Though it may be difficult at first to carve out this rest time from a busy schedule, it will pay back immeasurably in the long run in better health and fewer attacks. Yoga is based on nonviolence — to yourself as well as to others.

The compression and stretching exercises of Yoga will improve circulation, strengthen and stretch the chest muscles, and build a general sense of well-being. Compression poses are one of the most effective movements in Yoga because of their effect on increasing blood circulation to the vital organs such as heart and lungs, spine, nerves, and muscles. The exercises in the following routine are not strenuous and can be easily adapted for even less strain on the body.

Yoga breathing techniques strengthen and relax the muscles of your lungs. This will reduce the nerve activity in the airways, causing less constriction during an asthma attack. The Complete Breath exercise in particular can help during hyperventilation, and will increase awareness of your physical self. It will increase the capacity for personal observation, awareness, and change, and should be used before the meditation technique. It can also be practiced at any other times of day or as needed to prevent or alleviate an attack. The elasticity of the lungs declines somewhat as we get

older; however, we believe that regular daily practice of the Complete Breath will help keep the lungs elastic so there is no loss of respiratory function.

The relaxation and meditation technique will help you create a daily habit of rest and silence that will support you from within. The relaxation technique can also help during an asthma attack (see "Things You Can Do Throughout the Day," below).

• Special Concerns •

Difficulty in breathing can be serious; shortness of breath can signal other problems besides those related to the respiratory system. Consult a physician immediately if you experience any discomfort, and check with him or her about which exercises you should attempt.

When first learning the Complete Breath (Chapter 1), be careful not to exceed three repetitions at a time. If you haven't exercised your chest muscles in a long while, you may experience pain if you strain too much with the breathing exercise.

• Things You Can Do Throughout the Day •

When you feel an attack coming on, try these three steps to help relieve your symptoms and reduce your stress reaction:

1. Look for a quiet place to be alone.

2. Remember your complete relaxation procedure and use it to bring your mind into a more concentrated position.

3. Learn how to adopt a passive attitude. Consciously try to bring your body and emotions to a more quiet level.

If these three suggestions are followed, you can then begin to practice simple breathing and compression exercises that will gradually relieve your anxiety and improve your breathing. The compression poses (such as the Knee Squeeze, which can be done in a chair as well as on the floor or bed) will also help to reduce the panicky feeling of not being able to get your breath. Your relaxation routine may not remove all symptoms immediately, but it will help you greatly when you feel your symptoms coming on.

Most people do not consider a rest period in the day part of the regular day's routine. As a person with breathing problems, you should consider this part of your health regimen: give yourself a 15-minute quiet rest period every day in the middle of your work day. This can be done very easily by using your meditation technique during this rest period. You will have to find a suitable space that you can use every day. It may take some imagination, but it will be worthwhile in the long run, and you will look upon this place as a haven of rest from stress and anxiety.

• Dietary Suggestions •

Carefully check your intake of water. Try to drink at least six 8-oz glasses a day. This will help purify your system and encourage it to work more efficiently. Fluids dilute mucus.

Many times, breathing complications come from allergies, and some of the most common are allergies to food. You can check if this is a problem with an allergy specialist and avoid most of them. But if symptoms still continue, you should consider a very common allergy that many people are not aware of these days: coal tar. Coal tar is a food additive (primarily used in artificial colorings and flavorings) that has been added to the American diet only in the last 50 years. Coal tar can cause many asthmatic symptoms. You will have to carefully read every label on everything you put in your mouth, watch out for hidden artificial color and flavor in products such as toothpaste or medications, and try to use foods and drinks that contain only natural ingredients.

• Daily Routine for Breathing Disorders •

Start with the basic routine described in Chapter 1, then incorporate the special exercises in this chapter. These exercises have been chosen because they improve circulation by compressing the internal organs and stretching blood vessels, increase stamina, stretch and relax major muscle groups, help you practice stress management skills, expand the chest wall, and improve the quality of respiratory function.

If you don't have time to do a full routine, do at least three warmup exercises and three of the exercises in this chapter, and always do at least a few minutes of meditation. Best results will be obtained by practicing a little every day. Learn to do breathing exercises throughout the day. Remember never to leap up out of meditation; come out slowly.

Here is a list of the full sequence of techniques (including the basic routine):

Complete Breath, p. 26
Warmups, pp. 16-20 (Many of these exercises can be done in a chair.)
Arm Reach, pp. 60-61
Arm Swing, p. 61
Dancer Pose, p. 61
Standing Sun Pose, p. 21
Baby Pose, p. 24
Cat Breath, p. 62
Camel Pose, p. 62
Frog Pose, p. 63
Seated Sun Pose, p. 22
Tortoise Stretch, p. 23
Knee Squeeze, p. 63
Easy Bridge, p. 64
Cobra Pose, p. 64
Relaxation and Meditation, pp. 26-27

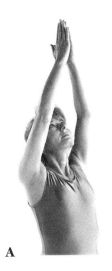

A

Arm Reach. *Limbers and releases tension in shoulders and upper back; improves respiration.* In a comfortable seated position (or standing), breathe out with your arms at your sides, then breathe in and raise your arms in a wide circle over your head (**A**). Look up and stretch. Breathe out and lower. Repeat twice more.

Arm Swing. *Limbers and releases tension in upper back; improves respiration.* In a comfortable seated position (or standing), stretch arms straight in front of you with palms together (**B**). Breathe out. Breathe in as you stretch your arms to the sides and back as far as possible without strain (**C**). Repeat twice more.

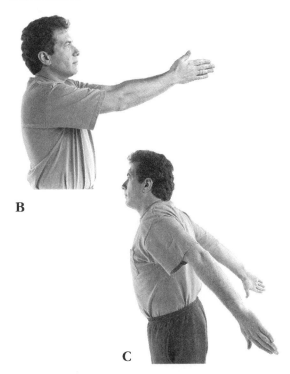

B

C

Dancer Pose. *Strengthens the lower back; limbers and strengthens the hips and thighs; improves mental poise; improves posture, balance, and concentration; strengthens ankles; relieves upper back tension.* Throughout the exercise, steady yourself by fixing your gaze on one spot on the wall in front of you. From a standing rest position, bend your right knee and grasp your right foot in back with your left hand (**D**). Check to be sure your stomach muscles are relaxed and your breathing steady. Slowly move into the completed Dancer Pose by raising your right arm straight up toward the ceiling so it is next to your ear and pulling your right leg up and back as far as possible without strain (**E**). Don't lean forward, and keep your supporting leg straight. Relax your stomach, breathe normally, and keep your gaze fixed on one spot. Hold for a count of three, then carefully return to the beginning position. [3 times each side]

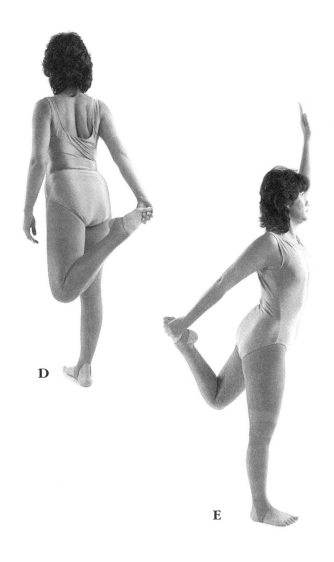

D

E

For more of a challenge: add the **Dancer Pose Extension**. Try this extension after you have become proficient in the Dancer Pose. From the Dancer position after your three-count hold as described above, maintain your gaze and, still breathing normally, slowly lower your body into the extended position (**A**). In addition to the benefits of the Dancer Pose, this variation stretches the back of the legs and increases strength and stamina. Keep your right leg as far up and back as possible. Your right arm extends straight ahead. Your left (supporting) leg remains straight. Stare at one spot for balance and hold for a count of three. Don't strain. Come back to a standing rest position.

Cat Breath. *Limbers lower and midback; tightens stomach muscles; improves breathing* Start on hands and knees. Breathe in, arch your back, and look up, so you feel the stretch all along your spine from tailbone to neck (**B**). Hold for a count of three. Then breathe out, round your back, and pull up on your stomach to increase the forward stretch (**C**). Tuck your chin and hold for a count of three. [3 repetitions]

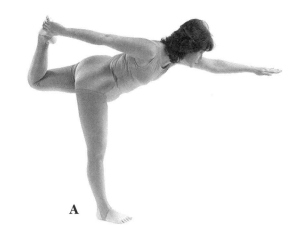

A

Camel Pose. *Limbers entire spine; improves circulation and respiration; stretches and strengthens thighs and knees; improves functioning of thyroid; strengthens heart.* Kneel with legs slightly separated. The first two movements in this exercise help to prepare the spine for an intense stretch: Carefully bend back and grasp your left heel with your left hand. Push your hips forward slightly (**D**). Repeat on the right side. Now bend backward and grasp one heel with each hand. Push your hips forward as far as possible and let your head relax back (**E**) (unless you have neck problems, in which case do not let your head drop backward). Hold for a count of three, breathing normally. As you get stronger, you can repeat if you wish. Release and rest briefly in the Baby Pose. [1 repetition]

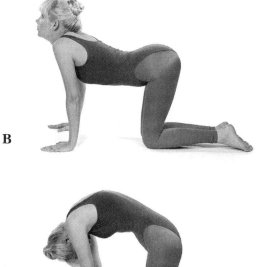

B

C

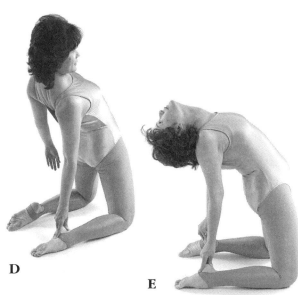

D

E

Frog Pose. *Limbers all respiratory muscles; limbers lower back and neck; relieves tension in spine.* Sit in a comfortable position on the floor with hips raised on cushions (see Chapter 1) or sit on the edge of a chair with feet flat. Place your hands on your knees. Breathe out completely and round your back, tucking your chin toward your chest (**A**). Hold for a count of three, then breathe in and arch your back forward, sticking your chin forward (**B**). Hold for a count of three. [3 repetitions]

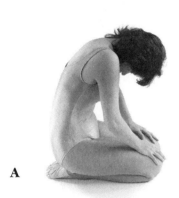

A

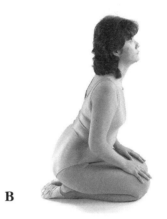

B

Knee Squeeze. *Improves digestion; limbers and relaxes lower back and hips; improves circulation in pelvic region; removes poisons from the body.* Lie on your back with arms over your head on the floor. Breathe out completely. Keeping your right knee straight, breathe in, bend your left knee, and lift your head, wrapping your arms around the knee. Hold your breath in and squeeze your knee to your chest (**C**). Hold for a count of three, then release, breathe out, and lower the leg and arms back to the starting position. [3 times each side, alternating]

After 3 repetitions on each side, do the same exercise lifting both legs at once (**D**). [3 repetitions]

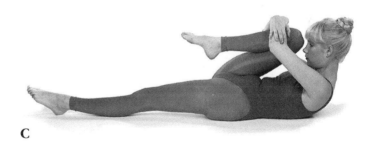

C

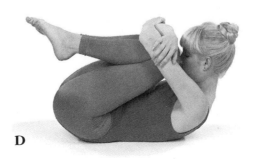

D

Easy Bridge. *Improves functioning of thyroid; eases back pain and fatigue; increases circulation to head; helps relieve bedsores.* Lying on your back, bend your knees and bring your feet as close to your hips as possible. Separate your feet several inches. Place your arms palms down at your sides (**A**). Relax your neck and upper back, breathe out completely, pushing your waist to the floor slightly, then breathe in and raise your hips, curling up just to your waist (**B**) (your back will be rounded and your chin tucked toward

your chest). Hold for a count of three, then breathe out and lower. Next, breathe in and lift your hips as high as you can without strain, keeping your shoulders on the floor and arching your back (**C**). Your chin will be tucked into your chest. Hold for a count of three, then slowly lower and breathe out. As you become more limber, you can hold on to your ankles for a greater stretch. [3 repetitions each variation]

Cobra Pose. *Improves functioning of digestive, respiratory, and reproductive systems; limbers and strengthens entire spine; strengthens eyesight; equalizes two sides of body; improves complexion.* Lie on your stomach with legs together (those with occasional lower back trouble should separate the legs at first). Place your forehead on the floor and your palms down next to your armpits close to your body so your elbows point back and up, not out to the sides (**D**). Breathe out completely, then start to breathe in as you curl first your head and eyes back as far as they will go, then your chest, and then your stomach (**E**). Keep your hipbones on the floor — this is not a push-up — and your arms slightly bent (unless you are extremely limber). Use your back muscles more than your arms. Hold for a count of three with your breath in and eyes looking up through your forehead. Do not blink. Then start to breathe out and curl forward slowly, in reverse: your stomach curls down first, then your chest, and finally your head and eyes. Your eyes are the first part of your body to curl up and the last to curl down. [3 repetitions]

Caution: This is a very powerful exercise and should not be done if you have had recent surgery or by women during the menstrual period, as it encourages blood flow.

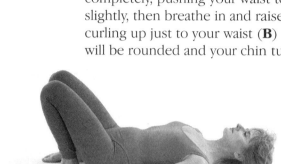

A

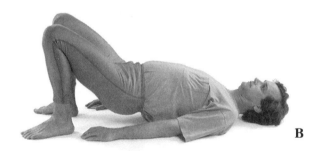

B

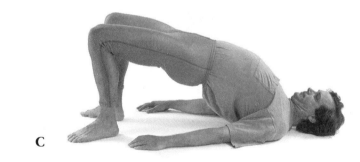

C

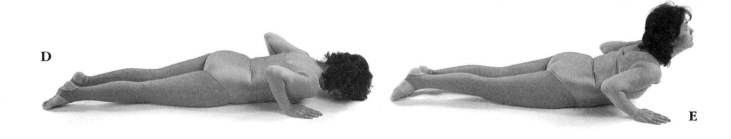

D

E

Yoga and Emphysema

In 1980 I was diagnosed with emphysema. At that time I had been practicing Yoga with the American Yoga Association for 10 years. In the beginning I accepted having this illness, but as time went on I decided to see if there were some way the practice of Yoga could help me. I signed up for a class on how to design your own Yoga routine for specific goals, and I worked out a routine to help me breathe better.

A few years later I took a trip to Kashmir where I roomed on the third floor of a house in the city of Srinagar. At first I had to stop for breath between every floor when going to my room. After a couple of weeks someone stopped me and asked if I had noticed how I was practically flying up the stairs! It was true, I did see a big change in my health and strength. And this in spite of the fact of living at high altitude (over 6,000 feet) in a city with extreme pollution — both reasons my doctor had advised me not to take the trip in the first place. When I returned to the U.S. I went for my annual physical where I took the same pulmonary tests I had taken for years. But this time the tests showed that my breath capacity had actually improved. In the 15 years that I have had emphysema, the condition has steadily improved. I take less medication than prescribed, and then only when I feel I really need it. I no longer fear being incapacitated by this disease.

— C. G., Yoga teacher and Director of Curriculum for the American Yoga Association

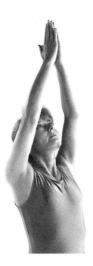

The Importance of Posture

To breathe correctly and completely, your spine must be straight. You don't have to sit on the floor in order to do breathing exercises; the edge of a straight chair is fine. You can even sit on the edge of your bed, as long as your feet are flat on the floor. In any position, your back will be most comfortable if your hips are higher than your knees. If you are sitting on the floor cross-legged, put a generously stuffed cushion under your hips. If your knees are stiff, you may need more than one cushion under your hips. If even this doesn't bring your hips higher than your knees, sit in a chair until your knees limber up. You can tuck your toes under the chair slightly in order to increase the tilt of your hips forward. When you are in the correct position, you will feel a slight arch in your lower back that will relax your entire spine. You will find that when you are in the correct position, you can hold it for several minutes without fatigue.

When you breathe, make sure your head and neck remain straight. Some people unconsciously bend their head and upper back forward as they breathe out and straighten as they breathe in. This decreases the effectiveness of breathing because it means you are using your spine to move the air in and out rather than your chest muscles.

Rest your hands on your stomach while you're checking the movement of the breath, or rest your hands on your knees. Do not let your hands fall into your lap, as this constricts the movement of the rib cage.

Chapter 6

Back and Neck

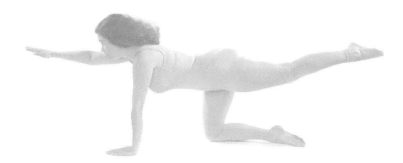

*N*ext to the common cold, back pain is the main reason why people see their physician. It is also the most common work injury. It is estimated that chronic back pain cripples over 2.5 million Americans each year, affecting all areas of their daily life. Victims often find themselves caught in a cycle of pain: the pain causes less activity, which leads to depression and withdrawal from normal activities, and the inactivity causes the pain to continue or even worsen. The most common area of the spine that is affected is the lumbar region, or the lower back.

Back pain stems from a number of causes; the good news is that many of them are correctable. Pain may result from a new injury or an improperly healed old injury. It may be caused by chronically poor posture, which results in weak abdominal muscles and puts excess strain on certain parts of the spine. A sedentary lifestyle is a major risk factor for back pain. Sitting for long hours at a desk or computer, especially with ill-fitting furniture, creates chronic muscle tension that, combined with weak muscles, can put unusual pressure on the discs. Back pain can result from chronically contracted muscles due to unrelenting tension and poor stress-coping skills; the muscles become fatigued, shortened, and more susceptible to sudden injury. A poor diet can contribute to back pain by undersupplying necessary nutrients such as protein, essential for repair of muscle tissue, and

calcium, which builds bone. An inflammation of the muscles and the sheaths that envelop the muscles may also cause pain.

As one set of muscles is getting flexed, the opposing set is being stretched. Overdevelopment of one set of muscles may push posture out of alignment and cause back pain. Problems with the muscles, ligaments, nerves, and joints of the spine are often interrelated. Improper muscle conditioning can also cause pain.

Disc problems usually cause the most severe pain. The discs start out as soft, fluid-filled pads that separate the vertebrae of the spine. The natural blood supply to the discs stops at about age 20; after that the discs begin a gradual degeneration and slowly become drier, flatter, and more susceptible to injury. If a weak or degenerative disc is subjected to sudden trauma, it may herniate (swell and push outward) and press on surrounding nerves. Occasionally it may even rupture. Pain from a herniated or ruptured disc may radiate down the arms and legs because of the pressure on surrounding nerves. Exercise programs such as Yoga that increase flexibility in the spine and increase the blood supply to the areas surrounding the discs will help the discs stay healthy and lubricated.

The key to avoiding back pain is to establish a back-care program long before a problem actually appears. Follow a sensible exercise program that includes flexibility, strength, and relaxation training. Learn effective stress-coping skills. If you are overweight, resolve to lose some of those pounds which strain your back muscles and put extra pressure on your spine. Adjust your environment as much as possible to reduce the likelihood of injury. Start by examining your chairs and tables at work and at home. A properly fitted chair allows you to rest your feet flat on the floor, provides support for your lower back, and has hydraulic motion and arm rests. When you are working at your desk or keyboard, your elbows should be at a 90° angle. Sometimes a small footstool helps. Your mattress should be firm but not rock-hard, and your car seat should have some support for your lower back.

If you do injure your back, see your physician. Usually, the first recommendation is to rest until the pain subsides and to allow spasms to relax and any swelling to decrease. However, prolonged bed rest can be harmful because it weakens the postural muscles and will reduce muscle strength and even bone mass in only a few days. Inactivity also reduces blood circulation which is so necessary to bring nutrients to the damaged tissues. Most authorities strongly recommend resuming mild activity as soon as possible to avoid loss of muscle tone. The Knee Squeeze exercise (see below), for example, can be done even in bed to begin the process of relaxing and stretching the muscles.

• How Yoga Can Help •

Many physicians recommend Yoga exercise as a way to gently stretch and strengthen back muscles for both prevention and alleviation of back problems. In fact, if you've had physical therapy, you'll probably recognize several Yoga movements. In Yoga, a strong, flexible back is very important for maintaining posture, for insuring that the nervous system pathways are strong and clear, for improving circulation to the body and brain, and for maintaining the erect posture necessary for seated meditation in intermediate practice.

Yoga exercises can be helpful both in preventing and in healing an injury. Many Yoga exercises gently stretch and strengthen the muscles in the hips, back, and legs; others improve muscle tone in the abdomen, which

supports the lower back. In most people, muscles on one side of the body are stronger than those on the other; Yoga exercises stretch and strengthen both sides equally. If you practice every day, you will soon notice more relaxed posture and a more fluid carriage, and your back muscles won't tire as easily. You'll also learn how to recognize tension in your back and neck muscles more quickly so that you can release it before the muscles become tight and sore. Yoga exercises cause the release of the brain chemicals called endorphins that are responsible for feelings of well-being; these chemicals also seem to act as the body's natural painkillers.

Breathing techniques and meditation training will teach you how to relax your body and mind at will and to recover faster from stress reactions. Relaxation exercises teach you to become aware of tension in your muscles and consciously relax them. By doing this regularly you will develop a better awareness of muscle tension and postural problems throughout your day, allowing you to ward off potential back pain before it develops. For beginning meditation, which is done lying flat so the spine can remain straight without strain, place a few cushions under your thighs and knees to release any pressure on your lower back.

By exercising carefully, and by practicing a simple routine of exercise, breathing, and meditation every day, you can help your back and neck become as strong and healthy as possible.

• Special Concerns •

If you have suffered an injury to your back or neck, begin with extremely gentle movements that do not hyperextend the neck or back in either direction. In a class, your instructor should modify the Yoga exercises for you to be sure you don't strain. Even if you have had back surgery, there will always be some movements you can do. Take this book to your physician and work out a suitable program for yourself.

See your doctor immediately if your back pain is accompanied by problems controlling your bowel or bladder, numbness in your groin or rectal area, extreme weakness in your legs, a high fever, or rapid weight loss — signals that back pain may be a sign of a more serious disorder. Pelvic infections, kidney stones or infections, prostate problems, and hip disease can sometimes cause "referred" pain to the spine.

• *T*hings You Can Do Throughout the Day •

If your work involves sitting or standing in one position, get up every now and then and move around. Do some bending and stretching exercises, breathe deeply, and walk around for a few minutes. At your desk, bend forward and rest in the Baby Pose (a variation you can do in a chair is described on p. 52). See pages 105 and 107 for other exercises that can be done in a chair (Frog Pose, Seated Knee Squeeze, Seated Twist).

• *D*ietary Suggestions •

A balanced, anti-stress diet with plenty of protein to help repair muscles will help your body recover from injury faster, and will help build reserves of energy to avoid further damage from stress.

• *D*aily Routine for Avoiding Back Pain •

Start with the basic routine described in Chapter 1, then incorporate the special exercises in this chapter. These exercises have been chosen because they improve circulation to the muscles, gradually improve spinal limberness and strength, improve posture, increase abdominal strength, relax and lengthen major muscles, and improve oxygenation of the blood through better breathing.

If you don't have time to do a full routine, do at least three warmup exercises and three of the exercises described below, and always do at least a few minutes of meditation. Best results will be obtained by practicing every day. Do all exercises at half capacity at first, until you are confident that nothing causes strain on your back.

Here is a list of the full sequence of techniques (including the basic routine):

Complete Breath, p. 26
Warmups, pp. 16-20
T Pose, p. 69
Standing Sun Pose, p. 21 (Do this exercise at half capacity and do not pull at the bottom of the movement until you are sure that the exercise does not aggravate your condition.)
Baby Pose, p. 24
Cat Breath, p. 69 (Do this exercise and the Arm and Leg Balance at half capacity and do not pull in the bottom of the movement until you are sure the movements do not aggravate your back condition.)
Arm and Leg Balance, p. 70
Seated Sun Pose, p. 22
Tortoise Stretch, p. 23
Knee Squeeze, p. 71
Easy Bridge, p. 71
Floor Stretch, p. 71
Easy Cobra, p. 70
Boat Pose, p. 70
Relaxation and Meditation, pp. 26-27

T Pose. *Strengthens legs and back; improves vigor; tones abdominal organs; increases concentration, memory, and mental poise.* Start by holding on to a sturdy chair or counter for support. Stand about three feet away from the support and lean forward, keeping your neck straight so you are looking at the floor. Breathe in, balance on your left leg, and raise your right leg in back parallel to the floor — or as high as you can (**A**). Staring at one spot on the floor, see if you can loosen your grip slightly on the support without letting go completely. When you are in position, hold for a count of three, then breathe out and relax. [3 times each side]

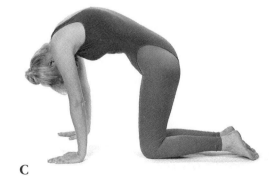

A

Cat Breath. *Limbers lower and midback; tightens stomach muscles; improves breathing.* Start on hands and knees. Breathe in, arch your back slightly, and look up, so you feel the stretch all along your spine from tailbone to neck (**B**). Hold for a count of three. Then breathe out, round your back, and pull up on your stomach to increase the forward stretch (**C**). Tuck your chin toward your chest and hold for a count of three. [3 repetitions]

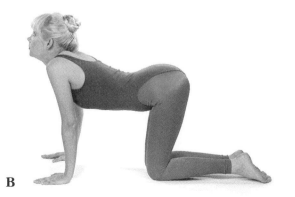

B

C

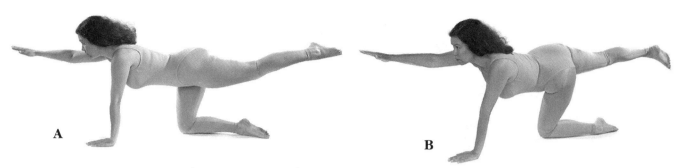

Arm & Leg Balance. *Strengthens muscles of the lower and midback, strengthens legs and hips; improves concentration.* On hands and knees, breathe out completely. Then breathe in and raise your left arm and right leg parallel to the floor (**A**). Look straight ahead at your outstretched arm, or, if your balance is shaky, stare at one spot on the floor. Hold for a count of three. Breathe out and lower. Repeat with the right arm and left leg. [3 each side, alternating opposites] If you feel very steady, you can vary this exercise by lifting the arm and leg on the same side of the body instead (**B**) [3 repetitions, each side]

Easy Cobra. *Gently limbers entire spine, balances both halves of body, improves circulation, massages all internal organs; helps increase lung capacity* Lie on your stomach resting on your forearms with hands clasped and elbows on the floor just below your shoulders, fairly close to your body. Breathe out and let your head and upper back relax forward (**C**). Now breathe in and lift your head and eyes up and back as far as possible without strain, then continue breathing in, arching your back and stretching up on your elbows, so you feel a slight stretch along your entire spinal column (**D**). Do not strain. Hold for a count of three and do not blink. Breathe out and relax your back, then your head and eyes, until your forehead comes back down to your clasped hands. Caution: this exercise should not be done if you have had recent surgery or by women during the menstrual period, as it increases blood flow. [3 repetitions]

Boat Pose. *Strengthens back muscles, improves digestion and functioning of all internal organs.* Lie on your stomach, forehead to the floor and arms stretched out in front. Breathe out, then breathe in and lift your arms, legs, and head (**E**). Look up. Hold your breath and the position for a count of three, then breathe out and lower to your starting position. [3 repetitions] If you are recovering from a back problem, begin by lifting only one arm at a time, then one leg, then gradually work up to lifting both arms, then both legs, and finally arms, legs, and head together.

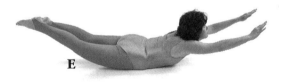

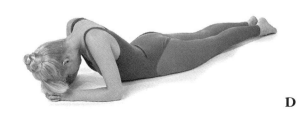

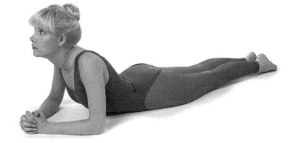

Knee Squeeze.   *Improves digestion; limbers and relaxes lower back and hips; improves circulation in pelvic region; removes poisons from the body.* Lie on your back with arms over your head on the floor. Breathe out completely. Keeping your right knee straight, breathe in, bend your left knee, and lift your head, wrapping your arms around the knee. Hold your breath in and squeeze your knee to your chest (**A**). Hold for a count of three, then release, breathe out, and lower the leg and arms back to the starting position. [3 times each side, alternating]

After 3 repetitions on each side, do the same exercise lifting both legs at once (**B**) (starting with knees bent instead of straight). [3 repetitions]

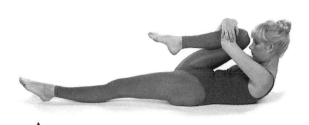

A

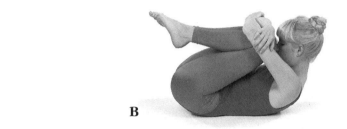

B

Easy Bridge.   *Improves functioning of thyroid; eases back pain and fatigue; increases circulation to head; helps relieve bedsores.* Lying on your back, bend your knees and bring your feet as close to your hips as possible. Separate your feet several inches. Place your arms palm down at your sides. Relax your neck and upper back, breathe out completely, pushing your waist to the floor slightly, then breathe in and raise your hips (your back will be rounded and your chin tucked toward your chest) (**C**). Hold for a count of three, then breathe out and lower. [3 repetitions]

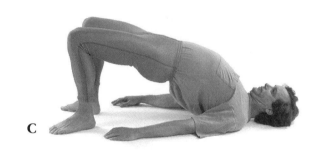

C

Floor Stretch.   *Limbers and releases tight muscles in entire spine and back of legs.* Lie on the floor on your back with arms overhead. Breathe normally. Stretch your left arm and leg in opposite directions, keeping feet flexed and pushing your heels away from you (**D**). Repeat on the right. Then stretch both arms and legs. [3 times each side]

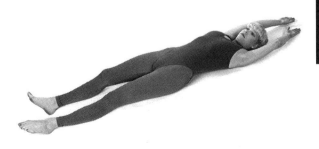

D

Chronic Fatigue Syndrome
Chapter 7

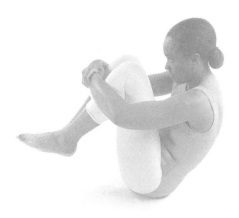

Chronic Fatigue Syndrome (CFS) burst into public consciousness in the 1980s, when it was at first somewhat derisively called "yuppie flu" or "affluenza" because it seemed to be most prevalent among young professionals. Since then it has been recognized as a very real, and very debilitating, disease of the immune system. Accordingly, there has recently been a movement to change its name to Chronic Fatigue and Immune Deficiency Syndrome (CFIDS).

In addition to the immune system, CFS affects the nervous, hormonal, gastrointestinal, and musculoskeletal systems. It usually appears with flu-like symptoms such as sore throat, fever, headache, and joint and muscle aches that don't go away in a few days as flu symptoms normally would. Its most evident symptom is extreme fatigue that comes and goes or lingers for long periods of time. Other symptoms include difficulty with concentration and memory, problems with balance, and sleep disturbances. CFS leaves some people bedridden; others can live a more-or-less normal life if they drastically curtail their activities. Most experience depression as a result of the constant debilitation and disability, and many experience periodic relapses that can be triggered by such factors as too much physical activity and weather changes.

It is not known exactly what causes CFS. Many theories are being considered, including heredity, environment, lifestyle, emotional stressors, sudden trauma, other illnesses, a head injury, anesthesia, or an allergic reaction. In the United States, those afflicted with CFS number in the millions. The disease is most likely to strike adults from their mid-twenties to late forties. The majority are women, and most are people with many interests and responsibilities.

Because no cure has yet been found, most doctors provide common-sense advice: Rest when you need it; eat a balanced diet; exercise at a level that does not increase fatigue; learn to pace yourself to reduce stress; learn what triggers a relapse for you; and adjust your lifestyle as needed to cope with your reduced energy level.

• How Yoga Can Help •

Contrary to most exercise programs that leave you exhausted, Yoga exercise leaves you refreshed and renewed, because it puts energy back into the system instead of draining it. When Yoga exercises are combined with breathing and meditation techniques, you will have a daily support system that makes a normal, productive life possible. One of my students with CFS was ready to give up her job as a stockbroker because of the debilitating effects of her disease. She found that a Yoga exercise routine every morning gave her enough energy to make it through the day, even in such a demanding profession.

Physical and emotional tension and fatigue lodge in muscle tissue, making it knotted, hot, and the circulation sluggish. Yoga exercises systematically stretch and relax the major muscle groups and push fresh blood and oxygen through the tissues, which releases tension and allows the muscles to relax and cool. The exercises are done slowly, and the breathing patterns with each exercise allow for maximum oxygen intake and for the release of toxins.

Poor circulation also means the brain and other vital organs get less blood and important nutrients. Yoga exercises improve all-over circulation by limbering the spine, by movements which improve elasticity in the blood vessels, and by selected inverted poses which use compression to pump more oxygen throughout the body.

Breathing techniques improve concentration and awareness, and help to reduce stress reactions. Extreme reactions to stress — especially when they are triggered by a past event or a future fear, or by a situation that cannot be changed — cause energy demands to increase rapidly. Your breathing techniques put you in touch with an unlimited source of energy that lies within you. By constantly returning the mind to the present moment, you allow the body to deal with what's happening now.

Relaxation and meditation conserve energy and build self-confidence. You learn how to relax every muscle in your body completely and then to forget about the body while turning your attention toward the mind in meditation. In meditation you simply stop all thought momentarily, allowing the strength within you to express itself. Meditation provides a refreshing, complete rest to the body and the mind.

People with CFS tend to ignore themselves. The "I Love You" meditation technique will help you build self-esteem and acceptance while you adjust to the lifestyle changes demanded by CFS.

• *T*hings You Can Do Throughout the Day •

Learn to use the Complete Breath to reduce harmful stress reactions and to recover more quickly from stressors. Do a meditation session at least twice a day to refresh and recharge.

• *D*ietary Suggestions •

Keep your energy level up by eating several small balanced meals throughout the day rather than three large ones. Emphasize foods rich in B vitamins and protein such as whole grains and low-fat dairy products. Fresh fruits and vegetables and legumes also help to improve the function of the endocrine system.

• *D*aily Routine for Chronic Fatigue Syndrome •

Start with the basic routine described in Chapter 1, then incorporate the special exercises in this chapter. These exercises have been chosen because they improve circulation and increase energy through compression of the body, stretch and relax major muscle groups through the use of "whole body" exercises, strengthen the respiratory system, and enhance mood.

If you don't feel strong enough to do a full routine, do at least three warmup exercises and three of the exercises described below, and always do at least a few minutes of meditation. Best results will be obtained by practicing every day. If you are unable to practice the entire routine at one time, do one or two exercises several times a day. Doing at least three exercises, plus three Complete Breaths and 15 minutes of meditation in the morning will give you the energy to see you through the day.

Here is a list of the full sequence of techniques (including the basic routine):

Complete Breath, p. 26
Warmups, pp. 16-20
Swing Stretch, p. 74
T Pose, p. 74
Standing Sun Pose, p. 21
Cobra V-Raise, p. 75
Baby Pose, p. 24
Hero Variation, p. 75
Seated Sun Pose, p. 22
Tortoise Stretch, p. 23
Knee Squeeze, p. 76
Easy Bridge, p. 76
Shoulder Stand, p. 77
Airplane Series, p. 78
Relaxation and Meditation, pp. 26-27

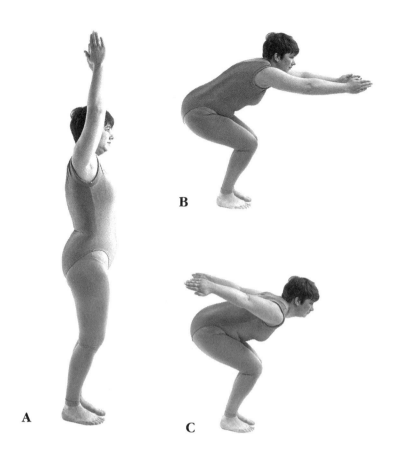

Swing Stretch. *Improves circulation; limbers the back and legs.* Standing with feet slightly separated and arms at sides, breathe in and stretch your arms forward and up as far as you can (**A**), then breathe out, bend your knees, and swing your arms down in front (**B**) and all the way back (**C**). Breathe in and swing back up with arms overhead, straightening your knees. Move with the breath. Stretch up as far as possible each time. [3 or more repetitions]

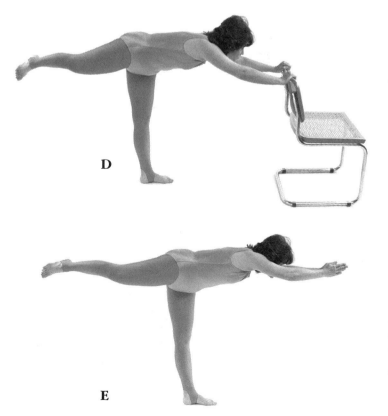

T Pose. *Strengthens legs and back; improves vigor; tones abdominal organs; increases concentration, memory, and mental poise.* Start by holding on to a sturdy chair or counter for support until you get more confident. Stand about three feet away from the support and lean forward. Balance on your left leg and raise your right leg in back parallel to the floor or as high as you can (**D**). It's important not to hold your breath in this exercise; let your breath relax; it will be faster due to the extra exertion required by this pose. Staring at one spot on the floor, see if you can loosen your grip on the chair. If you can, raise your arms straight in front of you and place your palms together (**E**). At first, keep your neck straight and look at a spot on the floor for balance. Later, you can try looking ahead over your two thumbs. When you are in position, hold for a count of three, then breathe out and relax. [3 times each side]

Cobra V-Raise.   *Strengthens legs, back, shoulders, and rib cage; strengthens heart; improves functioning of the organs in the pelvic region; reduces body fat.* Walk your hands forward on the floor, keeping your heels down as far as possible, until your hands are about 4 to 5 feet in front of you. Tuck your chin into your chest and breathe out. This is the "V" position (**A**). Now, keeping your arms straight, breathe in and slowly lower your body, arching your back and looking up and back (**B**) (the "cobra" position). Hold for a count of three. Push back slowly into the V position, breathing out and tucking your chin into your chest. Hold for a count of three. [3 repetitions]

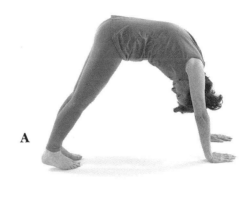

A

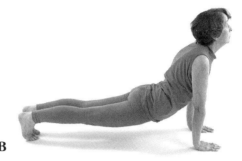

B

Hero Variation.   *Stretches rib cage; improves respiration and strengthens lungs; limbers upper back and shoulders.* In a kneeling position, clasp your hands in back and straighten your arms (**C**). Breathe in completely. Breathe out and bend forward, keeping your arms straight and pulled away from your body as much as possible (**D**). Hold for a count of three. Breathe in and come back up. [3 repetitions]

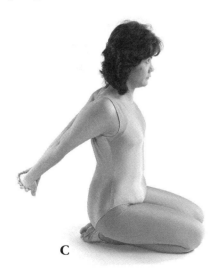

C

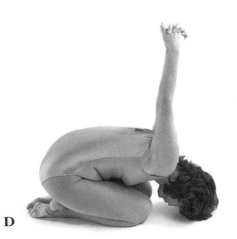

D

Knee Squeeze.   *Improves digestion; limbers and relaxes lower back and hips; improves circulation in pelvic region; removes poisons from the body.* Lie on your back with arms over your head on the floor. Breathe out completely. Keeping your right knee straight, breathe in, bend your left knee, and lift your head, wrapping your arms around the knee. Hold your breath in and squeeze your knee to your chest (**A**). Hold for a count of three, then release, breathe out, and lower the leg and arms back to the starting position. [3 times each side, alternating]

After 3 repetitions on each side, do the same exercise lifting both legs at once (**B**). [3 repetitions]

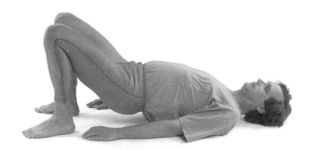

B

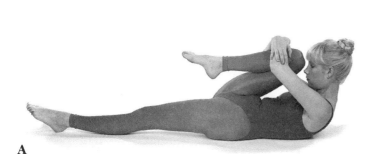

A

Easy Bridge.   *Improves functioning of thyroid; eases back pain and fatigue; increases circulation to head; helps relieve bedsores.* Lying on your back, bend your knees and bring your feet as close to your hips as possible. Separate your feet several inches. Place your arms palms down at your sides. Relax your neck and upper back, breathe out completely, pushing your waist to the floor slightly, then breathe in and raise your hips, curling up just to your waist (**C**) (your back will be rounded and your chin tucked toward your chest). Hold for a count of three, then breathe out and lower. Next, breathe in and lift your hips as high as you can without strain (**D**), keeping your shoulders on the floor and arching your back. Hold for a count of three, then slowly lower and breathe out. As you become more limber, you can hold on to your ankles for a greater stretch. [3 repetitions each variation]

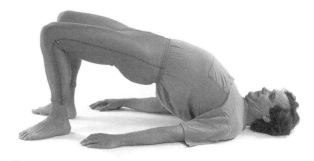

C

D

Shoulder Stand. *Stimulates thyroid and parathyroid; enhances function of all vital organs; relieves tension on heart and lungs; relaxes nervous system; removes fatigue.* If you have a disc problem in your neck, do not do this exercise; substitute the Easy Bridge (p. 76) instead. Start by sitting with knees drawn up to chest and arms wrapped around knees (**A**). Gently roll back and forth a few times (**B**) to make sure that the spine is in place with no pinched nerves or strained muscles. Then roll back, keeping knees to forehead, and immediately support your lower back with your hands and keep your knees bent and your body in the rounded position (**C**). Hold this position until you feel steady, then slowly straighten your legs toward the ceiling (**D**). If your legs appear to be more at a 45° angle, move your hands down your back toward the floor, push gently, and tuck your chin into your chest; your legs should straighten a bit more. Fix your gaze on the ceiling in the space between your big toes. Relax your breath. Hold for a count of three. As you get stronger, you can increase the hold to one-half minute, up to a full minute (do not exceed one minute). Women should not do this exercise during the menstrual period.

Come out of the pose by bending your knees and bringing them to your forehead. Cross your ankles (**E**) and slowly roll forward, rounding your back, until you come all the way up to a seated position. Bend forward for a few seconds to be sure the blood doesn't drain from your head too fast. [1 repetition]

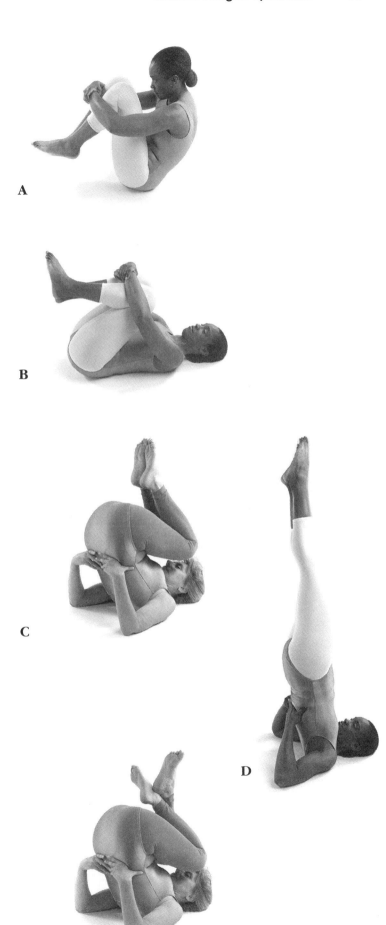

A

B

C

D

E

Airplane Series. *Strengthens entire spine; massages internal organs; improves breathing; strengthens shoulders, hips, and thighs.* This is a very challenging sequence but one which will give you a great deal of energy and strength. Lie on your stomach with arms overhead and forehead on the floor. Breathe in and lift your arms, legs, and head as in the Boat Pose (**A**). Hold for a quick count of three, then relax and breathe out, bringing your arms out sideways as in the Swan Dive. Breathe in and lift (**B**), holding for a count of three, then relax and breathe out, bringing your arms down to your sides. Breathe in and lift again (**C**), hold to a count of three, then breathe out and relax, clasping your hands behind you. Breathe in and lift (**D**), hold to a count of three, then relax and breathe out, grasping both ankles or feet. Breathe in and lift as in the Bow Pose (**E**), hold to a count of three, then relax and breathe out. [1-3 repetitions]

How to Make it Easier to Practice Daily

If you have trouble sticking to a daily schedule, or often feel too tired to exercise, try these hints for becoming more regular in your daily practice:

Wear the same clothing for exercise, and keep a blanket, towel, or mat separate to use only for Yoga practice. Once you've put on your Yoga clothes and spread out your mat, you've begun to create an atmosphere conducive to practicing. Another way to increase that atmosphere is to practice in the same room, at the same time every day. If you feel reluctant to exercise, tell yourself that you only need to do a few exercises, maybe just the warm-ups in Chapter 1. Then do those. If you still don't feel like exercising any more, don't force yourself. Lie down on your back, breathe deeply a few times, and then do a nice long relaxation and meditation session. Remember, it's not how much you do, but doing it every day, that will give you the best results.

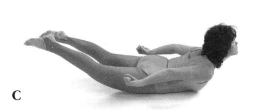

A

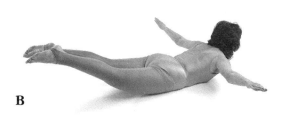

B

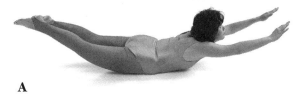

C

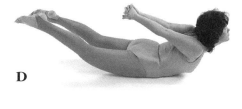

D

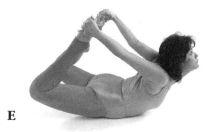

E

*E*veryone feels "blue" from time to time, but clinical depression — marked by persistent low mood, lowered self-esteem, and a loss of physical and mental energy — can be a serious problem. When depression persists for a long time, you may feel constantly sad, or you may feel nothing at all. You may have trouble eating and sleeping, leading to great fatigue. You may lose interest in sex and in other activities that used to make you happy. You may even experience hallucinations or consider suicide.

Some people feel ashamed of depression, seeing it as a sign of weakness and believing they should be able to "just snap out of it." Others think that if they just ignore their depression and suffer silently, it'll go away. And it may, for a while. But inevitably depression returns until the underlying problems are fixed. Left untreated, depression can suppress your energy for living, make you more vulnerable to disease by dampening the immune system, and even lead to suicide.

There are many possible causes for depression, among them changes in body chemistry. No one knows for certain which chemicals are involved, but depressed people seem to be deficient in certain chemical messengers. Depression might also appear due to genetic factors, or develop from a combination of too many psychological problems or traumas that the person is unable to resolve. Recent research has suggested that vulnerability to depression can be passed down in families through learned behaviors that include rigid thinking patterns, negative thinking, and self-defeating behaviors. Such inherited depressions often disguise themselves as alcoholism, addictions, eating disorders, and various psychosomatic complaints.

Major depression affects millions of people; it is estimated that about 10 percent of Americans will experience a serious depression in their lifetime. Men and women are about equally affected. The economic cost to society, in terms of lost productivity, permanent disability, depression-related drug and alcohol abuse, and the cost of treatment, is enormous. Research seems to indicate that we Americans are more depressed than our grandparents, perhaps a statement about our fast-paced modern lifestyle in which the pressure to perform and produce causes a great deal of unmitigated stress. The use of anti-depressant drugs is climbing rapidly, and the suicide rate among young women has increased 300% in the past 20 years. Unfortunately, only a fraction of those with depression seek professional help.

Depression is not all bad. Sometimes, the temporary pain and depression that come with growth and change in our lives is helpful, because it helps us see things the way they really are. It has been said that the world view of someone who is depressed is often more realistic than others who deny any "negative" or painful emotions. Many of us have grown up thinking that there is something wrong with us if we are unhappy.

• How Yoga Can Help •

Depression seems to be the ever-constant companion of illness and upset. It is talked about in flat tones with the hopeless qualities of a never-ending burden.

After so many years of Yoga practice and teaching, I am beginning to realize more and more that semantics has a great deal to do with attitude. I have discovered that many students have automatic negative associations with words like humiliation, depression, hopelessness, or fear. When I ask them to write a list of these words in one column on a piece of paper, and list what good comes from these things on the other side, they suddenly develop a new outlook. The old "lost in a well" feeling begins to balance out as they begin to realize that all feelings have worth; this is a new experience for them. Depression is a warning that may help you to protect your mental and physical health. Instead of just accepting it as a major blow to your life that means only sadness, try to balance this sadness with the realization that depression can be viewed as a signpost, signaling "It's time for a change."

The first thing a depressed person stops doing is moving. Regular exercise becomes intolerable. But Yoga exercise, starting with as few as three poses a day in just a few minutes' time, coupled with correct breath patterns, can become so pleasant to you that soon you will want to do more and more. The heavy, unmoving feeling of depression will be on the run! Yoga exercises put pressure on glands and organs, helping them to produce the soothing, healing chemical balance that is needed to feel well and be well. Yoga exercises improve circulation, sending invigorating oxygen to your brain and all your muscles. The stretching and strengthening movements flush toxins from the body as well.

Often depression sneaks in slowly, as breathing patterns change from too much sitting at a desk, stress, age, or illness. The deep, invigorating breath techniques of Yoga bring large amounts of fresh oxygen to the brain and other parts of the body. Like a spring wind, it blows through the system bringing new light and strength to the unused parts of the body and mind where depression hides.

Complete relaxation and meditation practice show you how to access the strength and power of your inner self for a support system that keeps you going through all the ups and downs of your life.

The best part of Yoga is its self-motivating quality. You will learn to help yourself through Yoga practice, and you will stay with it because it feels so good. Regular practice of Yoga will protect you from depression and help you stay bright-minded, while recognizing the signals that depression is giving you. To begin with, choose three exercises that appeal to you, and do them every day. Then, as you get more comfortable, expand your routine to give yourself more of a challenge and increase the beneficial effects. Do the "I Love You" meditation technique every day.

• Special Concerns •

Professional counseling can help you distinguish the harmful aspects of your depression from those that might be helping you in some way. Some therapies that are especially good for treating depression are cognitive-behavioral therapy and interpersonal therapy.

The use of anti-depressant medication is increasing at an alarming rate; unfortunately, medication is often handed out automatically — especially to women. Medication is necessary in some cases of very serious illness, and sometimes antidepressants or other drugs are the only way to adjust the body's biochemical balance so that a person can function well enough to begin using therapy and other treatments. If you are currently on medication for depression, you may wish to ask your doctor about alternatives.

• Things You Can Do Throughout the Day •

Do some exercise and breathing every hour. The Complete Breath and one or two simple stretching and bending exercises such as the

Full Bend Variation (p. 19) will fill your brain with fresh blood and oxygen and help to create a new outlook.

Practice the Laughasan exercise (p. 86) several times a day. This exercise is especially helpful in releasing endorphins that produce feelings of well-being.

• Dietary Suggestions •

Depression can be greatly helped by good nutrition. If you are fighting the lethargy and low self-esteem of depression, you may not feel like eating regular meals; however, your body needs nutrients more than ever. On "good days," stock up on easy-to-eat, nutritious meals such as soups and casseroles that you can freeze in small portions for those days when you can't face cooking. Be sure your diet is rich in protein and B vitamins: low-fat dairy products, legumes, and whole grains are the best sources. Enlist the help of a trusted friend to help remind you to eat.

Avoid artificial stimulants such as caffeine; it may give you a temporary "high" but will plunge you into a deeper "low." Sugary foods often act the same way by artificially manipulating your blood sugar levels. If you reach for sweets when you are feeling down, try to change your habits and have a protein drink instead.

• Daily Routine for Depression •

Start with the basic routine described in Chapter 1, then incorporate the special exercises in this chapter. These exercises have been chosen because they help you focus on the present moment, stimulate the release of endorphins, improve circulation throughout the body and brain, help enhance self-esteem, and improve oxygenation.

If you don't have time to do a full routine, do at least three warmup exercises and three of the exercises described below, and always do at least a few minutes of meditation. Best results will be obtained by practicing every day.

Here is a list of the full sequence of techniques (including the basic routine):

Complete Breath, p. 26
Warmups, pp. 16-20
Tree Pose, p. 82
Twisting Triangle, p. 82
Dancer Pose, p. 83
Windmill, p. 83
Standing Sun Pose, p. 21
Baby Pose, p. 24
Spine Twist, p. 84
Seated Sun Pose, p. 22
Tortoise Stretch, p. 23
Knee Squeeze, p. 84
Shoulder Stand, pp. 84-85
Cobra Pose, p. 85
Laughasan, p. 86
Relaxation and Meditation, pp. 26-27

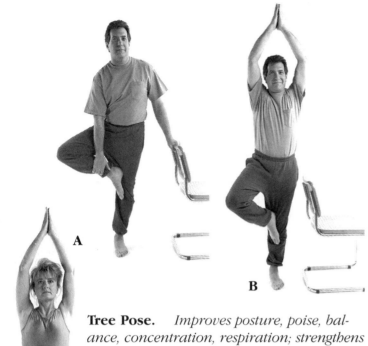

A

B

C

Twisting Triangle. *Increases flexibility and circulation in hips and lower back; strengthens hip joints and upper back; helps relieve depression.* Separate your feet as wide as you can comfortably (without losing your balance) and point your toes forward. Breathe in and raise your arms to the sides, parallel to the floor (**D**). Breathe out as you bend toward the left leg, grasp the outside of your left ankle (or calf) with your right hand, then turn your head so you are looking at your left hand, which should be pointed straight up, fingers curled and thumb toward you (**E**). Stare at your thumb. You can pull slightly with your right hand to increase the stretch. Keep both knees straight. Hold for a count of three, then breathe in and come back to your starting position, arms outstretched. [3 times each side, alternating]

Tree Pose. *Improves posture, poise, balance, concentration, respiration; strengthens legs.* Stare at one spot on the wall or floor in front of you (but keep your head straight). Breathing normally, slowly raise your right leg and place it as high on the inside of your left leg as possible (**A**). Position your foot so your toes point down, and relax the leg. Both these suggestions will help keep your foot from slipping down your leg. When you feel steady, exhale completely, then slowly breathe in and raise both arms over your head. Straighten your arms and place your palms together (**B**). Now relax your breath and hold the pose for a count of three. Watch for tightness in your stomach muscles which will tense your breathing. Relax your breath throughout. Keep staring at one spot for balance. If you have trouble balancing, practice this exercise standing next to a sturdy chair or the wall, and hold on with one hand. It's more important to relax your breath in this balance pose than to raise your arms overhead. If you are very limber and your back is strong, you may try the exercise with your ankle resting on the thigh (**C**). [3 times each side]

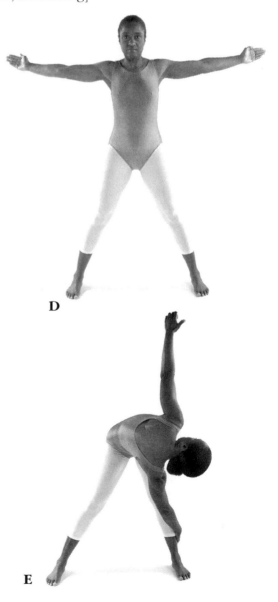

D

E

Dancer Pose.   *Strengthens the lower back; limbers and strengthens the hips and thighs; improves mental poise; improves posture, balance, and concentration; strengthens ankles; relieves upper back tension.* Throughout the exercise, steady yourself by fixing your gaze on one spot on the wall in front of you. From a standing rest position, bend your right knee and grasp your right foot in back with your left hand (**A**). Check to be sure your stomach muscles are relaxed and your breathing steady. Slowly move into the completed Dancer Pose by raising your right arm straight up toward the ceiling so it is next to your ear and pulling your right leg up and back as far as possible without strain (**B**). Don't lean forward, and keep your supporting leg straight. Relax your stomach, breathe normally, and keep your gaze fixed on one spot. Hold for a count of three, then carefully return to the beginning position. [3 times each side]

For more of a challenge: add the **Dancer Pose Extension**. Try this extension after you have become proficient in the Dancer Pose. From the Dancer position after your 3-count hold as described above, maintain your gaze and, still breathing normally, slowly lower your body into the extended position (**C**). In addition to the benefits of the Dancer Pose, this variation stretches the back of the legs and increases strength and stamina. Keep your right leg as far up and back as possible. Your right arm extends straight ahead. Your left (supporting) leg remains straight. Stare at one spot for balance and hold for a count of three. Don't strain. Come back to a standing rest position.

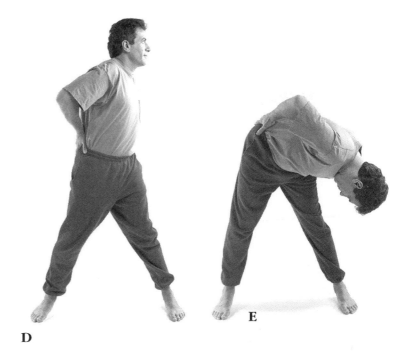

D   **E**

Windmill.   *Limbers and strengthens lower back, hip joints, and upper thigh; improves respiration; reduces waistline.* Stand with your feet as far apart as you can comfortably, toes pointed in. Place your hand on your lower back, thumbs over your hips and fingers supporting your lower back (**D**). Start by breathing in completely and turning toward the left. Breathe out as you bend your head toward your left leg (**E**) and continue moving over to your right leg. Now start to breathe in as you come back to a standing position and face front. Finish breathing in completely. Repeat twice more in the same direction. Your breathing pattern in this exercise follows the circular movement of your head: You are breathing out for two-thirds of the circle (from standing, over to the left leg, then to the right leg) and breathing in for the remaining third of the circle (as you stand up). [3 slow circles each direction]

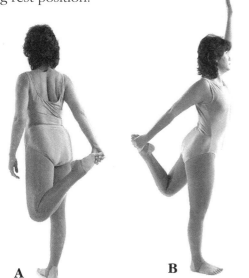

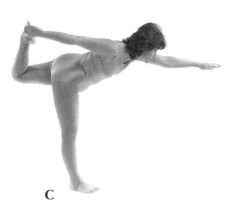

A   **B**   **C**

Spine Twist. *Improves digestion; limbers and tones entire spine; strengthens and limbers rib cage; relieves chronic constipation; helps relieve bladder, urinary tract, and prostate problems; strengthens heart.* Bend both knees. Rest your right leg on the floor, and lift your left leg over the right knee; the left foot should be flat (**A**). Sit up very straight, reach your right arm across your left knee, push the knee as far right as it will go, and grasp your left ankle; this locks the lower back into position (**B**). (Alternatively, if you are unable to reach your left ankle, grasp your right knee instead. You can also simply hook your right arm over your left knee and straighten the leg, as in **D**.) Now place your left arm behind you, straighten it and point the fingers in toward the base of your spine. Look forward, breathe in, then breathe out and twist toward the left as far as possible. Look far to the left with your eyes and stare at one spot (**C**). Hold for a count of three, breathing gently, and do not blink. As you get stronger, you can increase the holding time. Then release and slowly come forward. [3 times each direction]

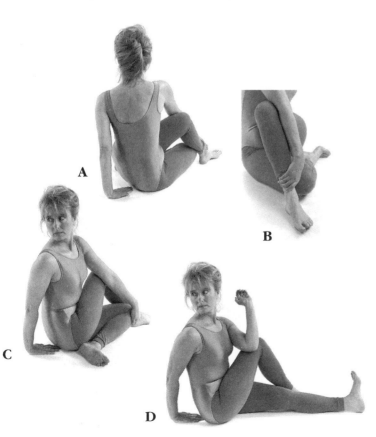

Knee Squeeze. *Improves digestion; limbers and relaxes lower back and hips; improves circulation in pelvic region; removes poisons from the body.* Lie on your back with arms over your head on the floor. Breathe out completely. Keeping your right knee straight, breathe in, bend your left knee, and lift your head, wrapping your arms around the knee. Hold your breath in and squeeze your knee to your chest (**E**). Hold for a count of three, then release, breathe out, and lower the leg and arms back to the starting position. [3 times each side, alternating]

After 3 repetitions on each side, do the same exercise lifting both legs at once (**F**). [3 repetitions]

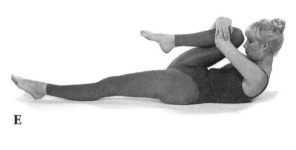

E

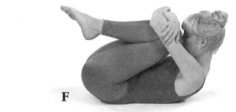

F

Shoulder Stand. *Stimulates thyroid and parathyroid; enhances function of all vital organs; relieves tension on heart and lungs; relaxes nervous system; removes fatigue.* If you have a disk problem in your neck, do not do this exercise; substitute the Easy Bridge (p. 92) instead. Start by sitting with knees drawn up to chest and arms wrapped around knees (**A**, next page). Gently roll back and forth a few times (**B**) to make sure that the spine is in place with no pinched nerves or strained muscles. Then roll back, keeping knees to forehead, and immediately support your lower back with your hands and keep your knees bent and your body in the rounded position (**C**). Hold this position until

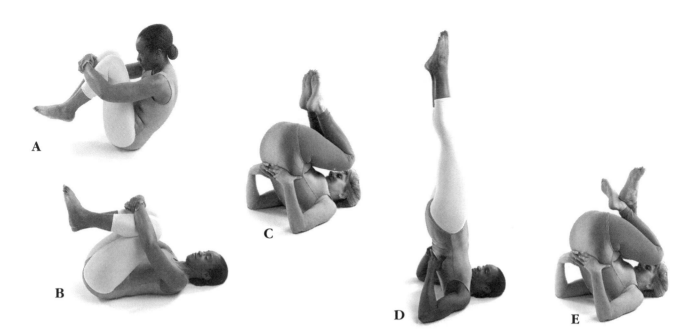

you feel steady, then slowly straighten your legs toward the ceiling (**D**). If your legs appear to be more at a 45° angle, move your hands down your back toward the floor, push gently, and tuck your chin into your chest; your legs should straighten a bit more. Fix your gaze on the ceiling in the space between your big toes. Relax your breath. Hold for a count of three. As you get stronger, you can increase the hold to one-half minute, up to a full minute (do not exceed one minute). Women should not do this exercise during the menstrual period.

Come out of the pose by bending your knees and bringing them to your forehead. Cross your ankles (**E**) and slowly roll forward, rounding your back, until you come all the way up to a seated position. Bend forward for a few seconds to be sure the blood doesn't drain from your head too fast. [1 repetition]

Cobra Pose. *Improves functioning of digestive, respiratory, and reproductive systems; limbers and strengthens entire spine; strengthens eyesight; equalizes two sides of body; improves complexion.* Lie on your stomach with legs together (those with occasional lower back trouble should separate the legs at first). Place your forehead on the floor and your palms down next to your armpits close to your body so your elbows point back and up, not out to the sides (**F**). Breathe out completely, then start to breathe in as you

curl first your head and eyes back as far as they will go, then your chest, and then your stomach (**G**). Keep your hipbones on the floor — this is not a push-up — and your arms slightly bent (unless you are extremely limber). Use your back muscles more than your arms. Hold for a count of three at the top with your breath in and eyes looking up through your forehead. Do not blink. Then start to breathe out and curl forward slowly, in reverse: your stomach curls down first, then your chest, and finally your head and eyes. Your eyes are the first part of your body to curl up and the last to curl down.
[3 repetitions]

Caution: This is a very powerful exercise and should not be done if you have had recent surgery or by women during the menstrual period, as it encourages blood flow.

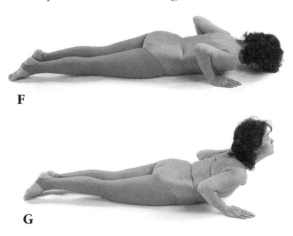

Laughasan. *Relieves muscle tension in the entire body; activates the immune system and releases endorphins.* Lie on your back and start pumping your legs as if you were riding a bicycle. Move your arms, too, and start to laugh (**A**). Pump your arms and legs as vigorously as you can and laugh out loud for at least 30 seconds. (This exercise can also be done in a chair.) Do this several times a day for a wonderful ebullient feeling.

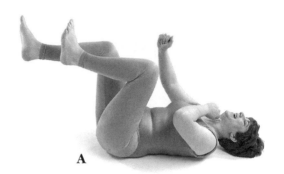

A

Yoga and Depression

Yoga techniques have helped me conquer the mental and physical damages from many years of clinical depression. The lethargy, fatigue, and pain associated with depression have left me. I look forward to the wonder every day brings instead of not wanting to get out of bed in the morning. I feel tremendous mental energy to fight any negative thought patterns that arise.

— J. M., direct care worker in mental retardation field, Cleveland, Ohio

Saying Good-bye to Prozac

I have suffered from clinical depression and anxiety attacks. I have tried coming off of Prozac two times, but was unsuccessful. And now I am completely off of all medication and I feel that Yoga (especially the breathing exercises and meditation) has been the key to my success. So I just thought I would share this with you and thank you.

— a college student in Cleveland, Ohio

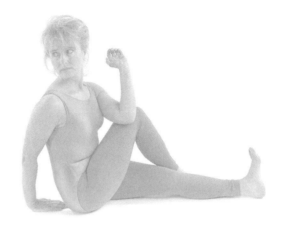

*D*iabetes is a chronic disease affecting many body systems and functions, particularly those concerned with metabolism. Type II (adult-onset) diabetes is less severe than Type I (juvenile) and is also the most common. About 90% of diabetics have Type II. Diabetes occurs more commonly among overweight people, women, the elderly, and the poor. The risk of developing diabetes increases as we get older. Heredity, diet, physical activity, race, and environment can also be factors in developing the disease.

Weight loss and regular exercise have both been shown to help in the treatment of diabetes as well as to help prevent its onset. Regular exercise has many other benefits as well, such as heart/lung conditioning, lowering of high blood pressure, improved insulin sensitivity, lowering of cholesterol, stress reduction, and improved blood vessel and muscle tone.

If you are diabetic, you are more vulnerable to developing other health problems such as infections, circulatory disorders, kidney trouble, heart disease, eye problems, and nerve disorders, so it is especially important for you to follow a healthy lifestyle, consult regularly with your doctor, and learn to take an active part in regulating your own health.

• *H*ow Yoga Can Help •

While Yoga cannot "cure" diabetes, it can complement the lifestyle changes necessary to keep diabetic symptoms in check or prevent their onset, and it can help you feel more in control of your health and well-being.

If you need to lose weight, Yoga can help build your concentration and willpower so that it's easier to stay on a weight-loss program (see Chapter 16). Yoga is self-motivating, making it easier to stick to a daily schedule. Yoga breathing techniques are particularly helpful because they teach you to focus on one thing — in this case, your smooth, rhythmic breathing — to the exclusion of everything else. In addition to strengthening your will, this practice also reduces harmful stress reactions and conserves energy so that more of it is available for living your life the way you want to. Learning how to cope with stress is important to anyone dealing with a chronic physical condition.

Yoga exercises gently tone and shape the body, improve posture and flexibility, and contribute to feelings of well-being. You will love doing it! Most Yoga exercises have a profound effect on improving circulation, especially to the extremities. They help keep the blood vessels elastic, and, combined with relaxation training, have even been shown to reduce high blood pressure in some cases. After you've practiced for a while, you can add more vigorous exercises to your Yoga routine to give you the additional benefits of some aerobic conditioning and increased muscle strength. Yoga exercises gently press on the body's glands and organs, resulting in positive effects for the digestive, endocrine, and reproductive systems.

By releasing muscle tension and enabling you to relax at will, Yoga relaxation training helps reduce the harmful effects of physical and mental stress. Daily practice of meditation reveals a quiet, restful, stable part of yourself that supports everything you do, and teaches you how to draw on these inner resources for optimum strength and health.

Coping with diabetes does not mean giving in to an "illness" mentality; by following your physician's instructions and changing your lifestyle, you can create a life that is full, happy, energetic, healthy, and balanced.

• S**pecial Concerns** •

If you haven't exercised in a long time, or if you have had diabetes for many years, you should begin your exercise program gradually and only after consulting with your physician. Take this book to your doctor and review the techniques to be sure they are safe for you. For instance, if there has been damage to the blood vessels in your eyes, you may have to avoid exercises that involve bending over or that call for more exertion. You may also need to take a stress test to check the condition of your heart.

• T**hings You Can Do Throughout the Day** •

Use the Complete Breath to reduce harmful stress reactions.

If you have a sedentary lifestyle or sit at a desk for most of the day, get up every hour or two and do some simple stretching exercises to get your circulation moving and to begin to breathe better.

• D**ietary Suggestions** •

If you have been diagnosed with diabetes, your physician has probably already recommended a diet plan for you or referred you to a dietician. A sensible diet will be the support for your new lifestyle. Be sure to take advantage of the latest information on diabetes and diet that is being offered to the public now through many hospital community education programs.

A public outreach program from the National Institutes of Health called "Do Your Level Best" is offering a free patient information kit on the importance of tightly controlling blood sugar levels; call 1-800-GET-LEVEL.

• D**aily Routine for Diabetes** •

Start with the basic routine described in Chapter 1, then incorporate the special exercises in this chapter. These exercises have been chosen because they improve circulation — especially to the extremities. They also help you develop greater concentration, teach you stress-coping skills, help to stabilize your metabolism, and tone and relax the large muscle groups.

If you don't have time to do a full routine, do at least three warmup exercises and three of the exercises described below, and always do the full relaxation procedure and at least a few minutes of meditation. Best results will be obtained from daily practice.

Here is a list of the full sequence of techniques (including the basic routine):

Complete Breath, p. 26
Warmups, pp. 16-20
Alternate Triangle, p. 89
Twisting Triangle, p. 89
Standing Sun Pose, p. 21
Cobra V-Raise, p. 90
Baby Pose, p. 24
Spine Twist, p. 90
Seated Sun Pose, p. 22
Tortoise Stretch, p. 23
Floor Stretch, p. 91
Shoulder Stand, p. 91
Easy Bridge, p. 92
Bow Pose, p. 92
Relaxation and Meditation, pp. 26-27

Alternate Triangle. *Stretches and strengthens muscles in the back, hips, and shoulders; compresses internal organs, stimulating metabolism; improves circulation to legs and feet.* With legs separated as far as is comfortable and toes pointed forward, breathe in and raise your arms straight out to the sides horizontally (**A**). Breathe out and stretch to the left, reaching down your left leg with both hands. Grasp the leg firmly and pull gently by bending your elbows (**B**) (if you can't bend your elbows, grasp higher on the leg toward your knee; it's more important to pull with your arms [to avoid straining your back muscles] than it is to reach further down your leg). Tuck your head and hold your breath out for a count of three. Breathe in as you slowly straighten and bring your arms back into the outstretched position. [3 times each side]

Twisting Triangle. *Increases flexibility and circulation in hips and lower back; strengthens hip joints and upper back; helps relieve depression.* Separate your feet as wide as you can comfortably (without losing your balance) and point your toes forward. Breathe in and raise your arms to the sides, parallel to the floor (**A**). Breathe out as you bend toward the left leg, grasp the outside of your left ankle (or calf) with your right hand, then turn your head so you are looking at your left hand, which should be pointed straight up, fingers curled and thumb toward you (**C**). Stare at your thumb. You can pull slightly with your right hand to increase the stretch. Keep both knees straight. Hold for a count of three, then breathe in and come back to your starting position, arms outstretched. [3 times each side, alternating]

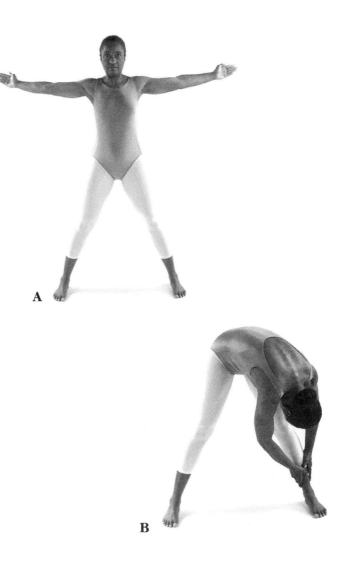

A

B

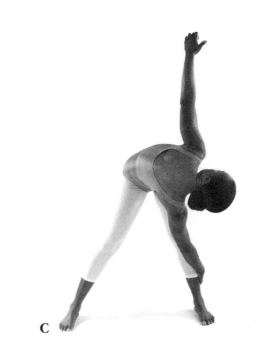

C

Cobra V-Raise. *Strengthens legs, back, shoulders, and rib cage; improves functioning of the organs in the pelvic region; reduces body fat; strengthens heart.* Walk your hands forward on the floor, keeping your heels down as far as possible, until your hands are about 3 to 4 feet in front of you. Tuck your head and breathe out. This is the "V" position (**A**). Hold for a count of three. Now, keeping your arms straight, breathe in and slowly lower your body, arching your back and looking up and back (**B**) (the "cobra" position). Hold for a count of three, and do not blink. [3 repetitions]

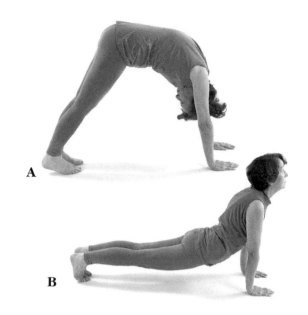

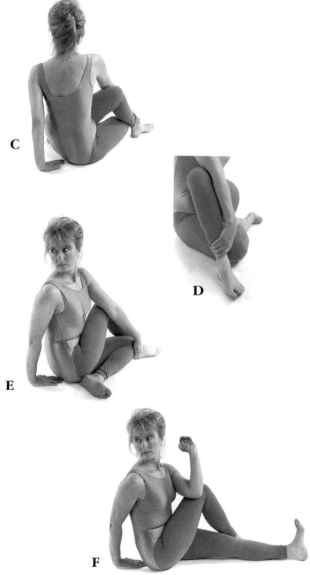

Spine Twist. *Improves digestion; limbers and tones entire spine; strengthens and limbers rib cage; relieves chronic constipation; helps relieve bladder, urinary tract, and prostate problems; strengthens heart.* Bend both knees. Rest your right leg on the floor, and lift your left leg over the right knee; the left foot should be flat (**C**). Sit up very straight, reach your right arm across your left knee, push the knee as far right as it will go, and grasp your left ankle; this locks the lower back into position (**D**). (Alternatively, if you are unable to reach your left ankle, grasp your right knee instead. You can also simply hook your right arm over your left knee and straighten the leg as in **F**.) Now place your left arm behind you, straighten it and point the fingers in toward the base of your spine. Look forward, breathe in, then breathe out and twist toward the left as far as possible. Look far to the left with your eyes and stare at one spot (**E**). Hold for a count of three, breathing gently, and do not blink. As you get stronger, you can increase the holding time. Then release and slowly come forward. [3 times each direction]

Floor Stretch.   *Limbers and releases tight muscles in entire spine and back of legs.* Lie on the floor on your back with arms overhead. Breathe normally. Stretch your left arm and right leg in opposite directions, keeping the foot flexed and pushing your heel away from you (**A**). Repeat on the other side. Then stretch arms and legs on each side, then both.

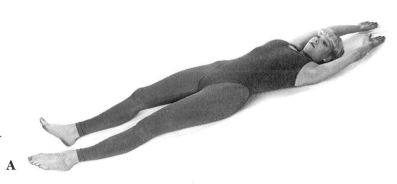

A

Shoulder Stand.   *Stimulates thyroid and parathyroid; enhances function of all vital organs; relieves tension on heart and lungs; relaxes nervous system; removes fatigue.* If you have a disk problem in your neck, do not do this exercise; substitute the Easy Bridge (p. 92) instead. Start by sitting with knees drawn up to chest and arms wrapped around knees (**B**). Gently roll back and forth a few times (**C**) to make sure that the spine is in place with no pinched nerves or strained muscles. Then roll back, keeping knees to forehead, and immediately support your lower back with your hands and keep your knees bent and your body in the rounded position (**D**). Hold this position until you feel steady, then slowly straighten your legs toward the ceiling (**E**). If your legs appear to be more at a 45° angle, move your hands down your back toward the floor, push gently, and tuck your chin into your chest; your legs should straighten a bit

more. Fix your gaze on the ceiling in the space between your big toes. Relax your breath. Hold for a count of three. As you get stronger, you can increase the hold to one-half minute, up to a full minute (do not exceed one minute). Women should not do this exercise during the menstrual period.

Come out of the pose by bending your knees and bringing them to your forehead. Cross your ankles (**F**) and slowly roll forward, rounding your back, until you come all the way up to a seated position. Bend forward for a few seconds to be sure the blood doesn't drain from your head too fast. [1 repetition]

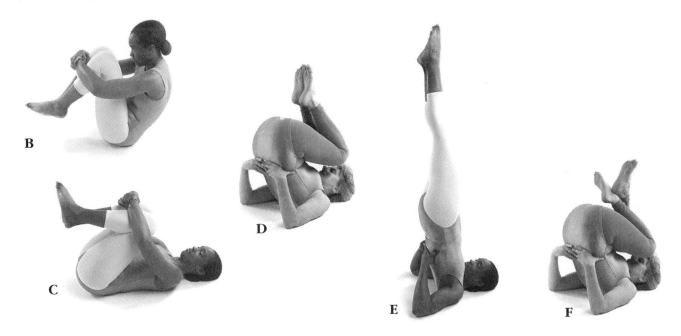

B

C

D

E

F

Easy Bridge. *Improves functioning of thyroid; eases back pain and fatigue; increases circulation to head; helps relieve bedsores.* Lying on your back, bend your knees and bring your feet as close to your hips as possible. Separate your feet several inches. Place your arms palms down at your sides. Relax your neck and upper back, breathe out completely, pushing your waist to the floor slightly, then breathe in and raise your hips, curling up just to your waist (**A**) (your back will be rounded and your chin tucked toward your chest). Hold for a count of three, then breathe out and lower. Next, breathe in and lift your hips as high as you can without strain, keeping your shoulders on the floor and arching your back (**B**). Your chin will be tucked into your chest. Hold for a count of three, then slowly lower and breathe out. As you become more limber, you can hold onto your ankles for a greater stretch. [3 repetitions each variation]

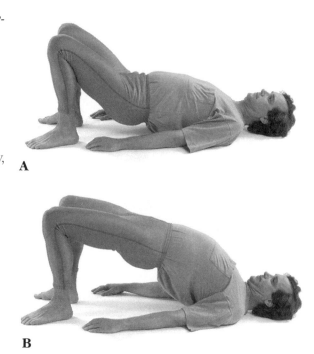

A

B

Bow Pose. *Relieves chronic constipation; improves functioning of digestive system; strengthens back and thigh muscles; increases vitality.* Lie on your stomach with your forehead on the floor and your knees bent. Reach back and grasp your ankles (**C**). Breathe out completely, then breathe in and lift up, balancing on your stomach (**D**). Look up. Hold for a count of three. Breathe out and lower to the starting position. [3 repetitions]

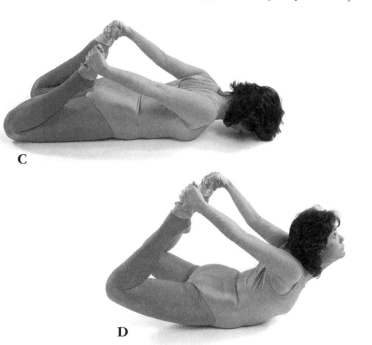

C

D

Details, Details

Doing an exercise perfectly in Yoga does not mean doing it with the greatest flexibility or strength, but with the most attention to detail. In most exercise programs, it doesn't really matter where you place your feet, or the position of your fingers, or where your gaze is directed. In Yoga, these details make the difference between a really effective technique and one where you are just going through the motions. For example, one of the important functions of Yoga exercise is to improve circulation. Especially with regard to diabetes, where circulation to the extremities is so important, you need to pay attention to the exercise instructions and be sure your hands and feet are in the proper positions. Occasionally an exercise instruction directs you to stare at one spot without blinking. This strengthens eyesight and improves concentration. The most important aspect of every exercise is its particular breathing pattern. Each exercise pushes the breath in a slightly different way, which improves oxygenation of the blood, flushes toxins from the muscles, and brings nutrients to the brain. Even if you do only a few exercises every day, make them perfect with regard to attention to detail.

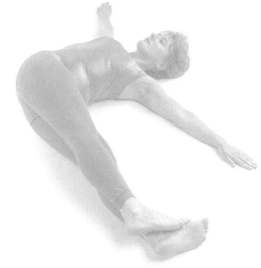

*E*ven if you suffer from headaches only infrequently, they can dramatically disrupt your life. While some headaches may subside within a short time, throbbing migraines can cripple individuals for days, and intensely painful cluster headaches may recur for days or even weeks. Tension headaches, while more common and usually less severe, also reduce productivity and can strain interpersonal relationships.

The pain of headaches can stem from several causes, including 1) overcontraction or tightening of the muscles of the head, scalp, face, jaw, or neck; 2) changes in the fluid pressure within the skull; 3) changes in the blood vessels of the head, scalp, face, jaw, or neck; 4) chemical changes, such as blood sugar or hormonal fluctuations, or allergic responses, especially from certain foods; 5) pinched nerves or other spinal or nervous system problems; and 6) TMJ syndrome (tightening of the temporomandibular joint in the jaw).

There are two main types of headaches: tension headaches and migraines. Tension headaches, also known as muscle-contraction headaches, account for approximately 90 percent of headaches and are the ones most likely to be caused by stress. Muscle contraction from chronic stress may cause the bones of the skull to become jammed, which may in turn result in pinched nerves, disruption of the endocrine system of the body, and/or reduced blood flow to the brain.

The body is one integral unit, and any imbalance in it can lead to a headache. However, certain muscles are most frequently involved in headaches: (1) The temporalis stretches from the temples down the front of the ear to the jaw. This can cause a headache upon awakening; to avoid this, do relaxation exercises before you go to sleep. Many people also tighten the jaw in stressful situations during the day; (2) The frontalis muscle is in the region of the forehead and the front of the head; it often tenses during periods of stress or deep concentration; (3) The occipitalis muscle is located at the lower back of the head; (4) The large trapezius muscles begin at the base of the skull and extend out over the shoulders and down each side of the spine. Overcontraction of these muscles can affect the vertebrae, irritating the nerves. Trapezius muscles can be chronically tense due to work conditions, living habits, bad posture, and stress. All these muscle groups can be relaxed through Yoga exercise, breathing, and relaxation techniques.

During stress, blood flow shifts away from certain organs, including the digestive tract, which can contribute to food allergies and toxicity, another frequent cause of headaches. Learning and using stress-management techniques will help prevent this type of headache. Deficiencies of certain nutrients such as protein or calcium can also precipitate a headache.

Migraine is the second major type of headache, and its pain comes from dilation of blood vessels which then press on cranial nerves. Approximately 18 million people in the United States suffer from migraines: three times as many women as men. Migraines can be triggered by such factors as too much or too little sleep, certain chemicals or medications, weather changes, flickering lights, exercise, sex, high altitudes, eyestrain, poor air circulation, and certain foods.

Hormone imbalances due to menstruation, pregnancy, heredity, a sluggish liver, or other causes may also contribute to migraine headaches, as well as possibly some dietary deficiencies such as a lack of adequate calcium and magnesium or protein. Migraine sufferers seem to have lower endorphin levels (the brain chemical which causes feelings of pleasure and acts as a natural painkiller). A recent study also found that migraine sufferers were more likely to have a history of anxiety and depression, which correlates with the theories regarding lower levels of endorphins. Two of the things that are known to raise endorphin levels are laughter and exercise.

• *H*ow Yoga Can Help •

Simple Yoga techniques can serve as an alternative or supplement to other remedies for dealing with headaches, as both prevention and treatment.

Tension headaches often can be prevented by regular attention to your body's state of tension: every hour or so, do some simple stretching, bending, and breathing exercises to keep your circulation moving, improve blood and oxygen flow to the brain, reduce any tension that may be building in your muscles, and flush toxins from the body. Some simple exercises can even be practiced at work (standing or in a chair) to ease tension that may cause a headache.

A regular daily Yoga session may help to prevent or reduce the number and severity of migraines as well. Regular exercise, breathing, and meditation will increase endorphins, build resistance to stress, strengthen your immune system, and help stabilize metabolism.

(Note: during a severe headache, especially a migraine, exercise often worsens the pain.)

A mild headache can often be alleviated by practicing deep breathing and relaxation in a lying-down position in a quiet place. Often this will be enough to relax tense muscles and return blood vessels to their normal size. Be aware, though, that the ability to achieve a relaxed state of mind — especially when you're in pain — takes practice. A daily Yoga routine that includes exercise, breathing, and meditation will help you learn and master the skills needed to relieve a headache. Another very beneficial technique is the Laughasan exercise (see below).

Yoga helps to increase self-awareness, enabling you to notice and take care of physical symptoms before they become severe. Breathing techniques help you cope with stress by conserving energy and helping you reduce harmful reactions. Meditation teaches you how to relax at will; during relaxation, the nervous system slows down, yet blood flow to the brain is increased. At the same time, you learn to enjoy new feelings of restful quiet.

• *S*pecial Concerns •

Persistent or severe headaches can sometimes be a symptom of an underlying medical problem. Be sure to consult your physician.

• *T*hings You Can Do Throughout the Day •

Mini-facial relaxation: Since many muscle-contraction headaches start with the small muscles around your face and neck, check and relax those places throughout the day. Close your eyes and apply a very light tugging pressure upward with your fingers to the two spots about three inches above your eyes. Hold for a minute or two, then release. Using your palms, lightly massage your temples, your jaw, and your neck. Do the Lion Pose and the Laughasan (below).

Do everything you can to improve your stress-coping skills. When you notice tension beginning to develop, take some time out. Do some Complete Breaths, a few stretching exercises that require you to breathe deeply, such as the Standing Sun Pose, and a ten-minute deep relaxation and meditation. It may be especially helpful for you to use a meditation tape (see Resources).

Check your posture every hour: chronic tension can develop in the neck muscles if you stand or sit with your chin jutting forward. If you notice yourself doing this, consciously lengthen the back of your neck and pull your chin back. Lift the top of your head straight toward the ceiling. Do the Neck Stretch exercise and the Standing Reach (see Chapter 1).

Try to notice the things that trigger a headache for you: keep a record of how you felt, what you were doing, what you ate, and where you were just before you developed a headache. Keep a record of how many times you laughed during the day.

• Dietary Suggestions •

Substances that are common headache triggers are aged cheese, chocolate, citrus, MSG, red wine, nitrites, caffeine, and aspartame. Some people also develop allergies to artificial color and flavor, or other artificial substances. Learn to read labels to avoid artificial food.

Since low blood sugar can contribute to a headache, it's important to eat regular, balanced meals. Make sure your meals are high in protein, and build protein snacks into your schedule. Also, be sure you are getting adequate calcium and magnesium. Women are especially lacking in these vital nutrients and often should consider supplementation. Some have found headache relief by taking a low dosage of calcium/magnesium every two hours throughout the day during the week or two just prior to menstruation when calcium levels drop precipitously — but be sure to consult your physician first, since some medical conditions may be worsened with excessive supplementation.

• Daily Routine for Headaches •

Start with the basic routine described in Chapter 1, then incorporate the special exercises in this chapter. These exercises have been chosen because they improve circulation, help to stabilize metabolism, compress internal glands and organs to stimulate hormone production, teach stress-coping skills, and release muscle tension.

If you don't have time to do a full routine, do at least three warmup exercises and three of the exercises described below, and always do the full complete relaxation procedure and at least a few minutes of meditation. Best results will be obtained by practicing every day. Since schedule changes can sometimes trigger headaches, try to do your Yoga routine at the same time every day.

Here is a list of the full sequence of techniques (including the basic routine):

Complete Breath, p. 26
Sitali Breath, p. 96
Alternate Nostril Breath, p. 96
Warmups, pp. 16-20
Standing Sun Pose, p. 21
Baby Pose, p. 24
Lion Pose, p. 96
Cat Breath, p. 97
Spine Twist, p. 97
Seated Sun Pose, p. 22
Tortoise Stretch, p. 23
Knee Squeeze, p. 98
Pelvic Twist, p. 98
Bow Pose, p. 99
Cobra Pose, p. 99
Relaxation and Meditation, pp. 26-27
Laughasan, p. 100

The following two breathing exercises can be done on the floor in a comfortable seated position or on the edge of a chair. If you sit on the floor, place a few pillows under your hips to take any strain off your lower back.

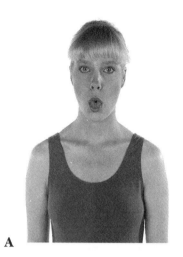

A

Sitali Breath. *Clarifies the nervous system by removing mucus from the nervous system.* Breathe out completely through your nose. Curl both sides of your tongue in toward the center and breathe in completely through your mouth (**A**). Hold for a count of three. Uncurl your tongue and breathe out through your nose. Hold for a count of three. Repeat several times, breathing smoothly and as slowly as you can without straining.

Alternate Nostril Breath. *Balances both sides of body; improves concentration; strengthens respiration.* Using your right hand, curl your first and second fingers in toward your palm and hold them with the fleshy part of your thumb. Extend the fourth and fifth fingers straight. Start by closing your right nostril with your thumb and breathe in through your left nostril (**B**). Breathe completely and slowly, just as in the Complete Breath. Then close your left nostril with the fourth and fifth fingers (**C**), and breathe out through your right nostril. Breathe in through the right nostril, then close with your thumb and breathe out, then in, through your left nostril. Continue for about 5 breath cycles to start (later you can add more repetitions if you wish). Focus on the sound of the breath. Breathe evenly and smoothly.

During a period when I experienced migraine headaches, I found it very helpful to do this breathing exercise first thing in the morning. Simply swing your legs to the floor, sit on the edge of your bed, and do a few cycles of this breath exercise before doing anything else.

Lion Pose. *Relaxes facial muscles; relieves anxiety and depression; changes mood.* Sit comfortably with hands on your knees. Take a deep breath in, then breathe out quickly with a growling sound as you open your eyes and mouth wide, stick out your tongue, and tense your fingers (**D**). [3 repetitions — or as needed]

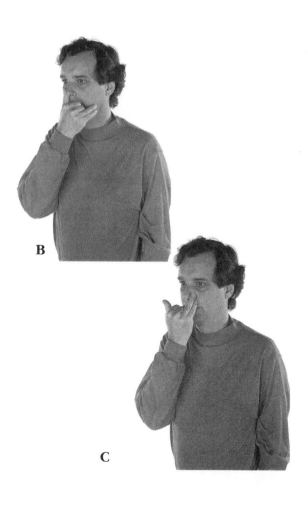

D

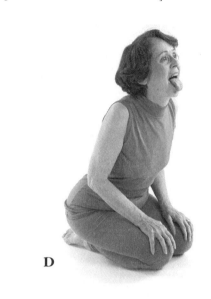

B

C

Cat Breath. *Limbers lower and midback; tightens stomach muscles; improves breathing.* Start on hands and knees. Breathe in, arch your back, and look up (**A**), so you feel the stretch all along your spine from tailbone to neck. Hold for a count of three. Then breathe out, round your back, and pull up on your stomach to increase the forward stretch (**B**). Tuck your chin and hold for a count of three. [3 repetitions]

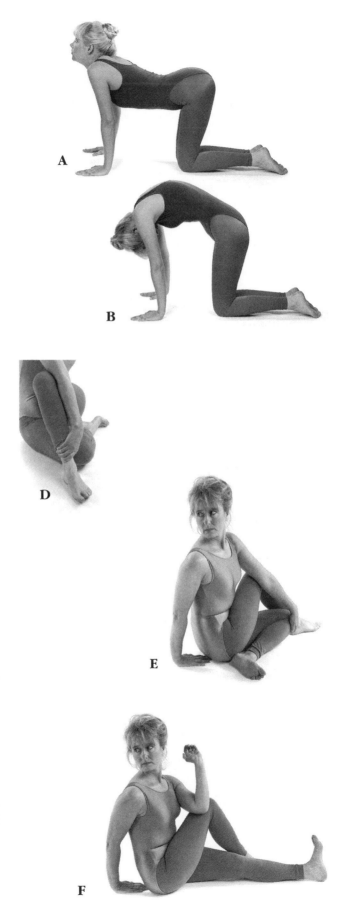

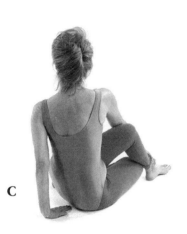

Spine Twist. *Improves digestion; limbers and tones entire spine; strengthens and limbers rib cage; relieves chronic constipation; helps relieve bladder, urinary tract, and prostate problems; strengthens heart.* Bend both knees. Rest your right leg on the floor, and lift your left leg over the right knee; the left foot should be flat (**C**). Sit up very straight, reach your right arm across your left knee, push the knee as far right as it will go, and grasp your left ankle; this locks the lower back into position (**D**). (Alternatively, if you are unable to reach your left ankle, grasp your right knee instead. You can also simply hook your right arm over your left knee and straighten the leg, as in **F**.) Now place your left arm behind you, straighten it and point the fingers in toward the base of your spine. Look forward, breathe in, then breathe out and twist toward the left as far as possible (**E**). Look far to the left with your eyes and stare at one spot. Hold for a count of three, breathing gently, and do not blink. As you get stronger, you can increase the holding time. Then release and slowly come forward. [3 times each direction]

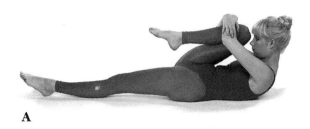

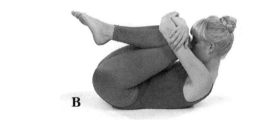

A

B

Pelvic Twist. *Compresses internal organs, stimulating circulation and metabolism; reduces waistline; strengthens lower back and legs.* Lie on your back with your arms outstretched, palms down. Bend your knees and bring them up toward your chest (**C**). This is your starting position. Breathe in as you slowly swing your legs toward the left as far as possible (keep knees bent). Hold for a count of three, then breathe out as you lift your legs back to your starting position. Breathe in and swing them to the opposite side. Hold for a count of three. [3 on each side, alternating]

After you've practiced this for several weeks, and if you have no back or neck problems, try a more difficult variation: when you swing your legs to the side, straighten them as they reach the ground (**D**), then bend them as they come back up to your starting position. The breathing pattern is the same. [3 each side, alternating]

Knee Squeeze. *Improves digestion; limbers and relaxes lower back and hips; improves circulation in pelvic region; removes poisons from the body.* Lie on your back with arms over your head on the floor. Breathe out completely. Keeping your right knee straight, breathe in, bend your left knee, and lift your head, wrapping your arms around the knee. Hold your breath in and squeeze your knee to your chest (**A**). Hold for a count of three, then release, breathe out, and lower the leg and arms back to the starting position. [3 times each side, alternating]

After 3 repetitions on each side, do the same exercise lifting both legs at once (**B**). [3 repetitions]

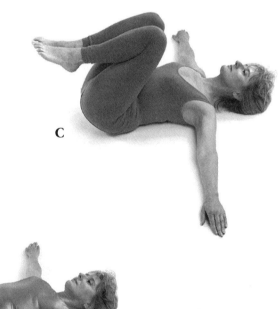

C

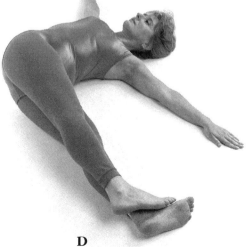

D

Bow Pose. *Relieves chronic constipation; improves functioning of digestive system; strengthens back and thigh muscles; increases vitality.* Lie on your stomach with your forehead on the floor and your knees bent. Reach back and grasp your feet or ankles. Breathe out completely, then breathe in and lift up, balancing on your stomach (**A**). Look up. Hold for a count of three. Breathe out and lower to the starting position. [3 repetitions]

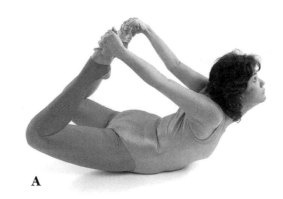

A

Cobra Pose. *Improves functioning of digestive, respiratory, and reproductive systems; limbers and strengthens entire spine; strengthens eyesight; equalizes two sides of body; improves complexion.* Lie on your stomach with legs together (those with occasional lower back trouble should separate the legs at first). Place your forehead on the floor and your palms down next to your armpits close to your body so your elbows point back and up, not out to the sides (**B**). Breathe out completely, then start to breathe in as you curl first your head and eyes back as far as they will go, then your chest, and then your stomach (**C**). Keep your hipbones on the floor — this is not a push-up — and your arms slightly bent (unless you are extremely limber). Use your back muscles more than your arms. Hold for a count of three at the top with your breath in and eyes looking up through your forehead. Do not blink. Then start to breathe out and curl forward slowly, in reverse: your stomach curls down first, then your chest, and finally your head and eyes. Your eyes are the first part of your body to curl up and the last to curl down. [3 repetitions]

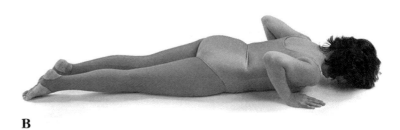

B

Caution: This is a very powerful exercise and should not be done if you have had recent surgery or by women during the menstrual period, as it encourages blood flow.

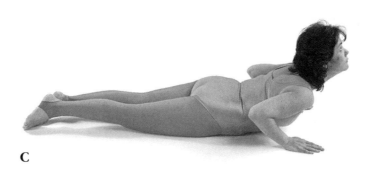

C

Laughasan.   *Relieves muscle tension in the entire body; activates the immune system and releases endorphins.* Lie on your back and start pumping your legs as if you were riding a bicycle. Move your arms, too, and start to laugh (**A**). Pump your arms and legs as vigorously as you can and laugh out loud for at least 30 seconds. (This exercise can also be done in a chair.) Do this several times a day for a wonderful ebullient feeling.

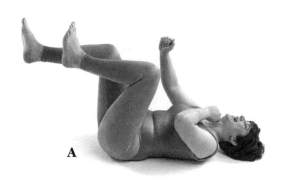

A

Hints for Balanced Breathing

When you sit to do breathing exercises, you may notice that one side of your nose is blocked; this is especially problematic for the Alternate Nostril Breath. To make both sides of your nose breathe evenly, make a fist with your hand and press into the armpit of the side on which you are breathing freely. For example, if your left nostril is blocked, make a fist with your left hand and press into the right armpit. Hold for several seconds or until the left side begins to clear.

Another technique that works to bring balance and clarity to your whole day is to pay attention to your breathing when you get out of bed. When you stand up, step first on the foot that is on the same side as the nostril that is open; that is, if your left side is blocked, step first on the right foot.

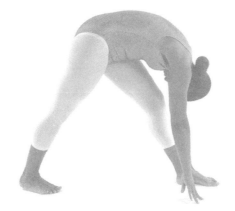

*T*he cardiovascular system is responsible for the important tasks of delivering oxygen and nutrients to your body's organs and removing waste products from the cells. The oxygen and nutrients transported in the bloodstream and delivered with each beat of the heart nourish 300 trillion cells. The heart never rests, except for a split second between beats, and it works up to ten times as hard during exercise or stress as it does at rest. Obviously, a stronger muscle works more efficiently. The heart muscle weakens through disuse (lack of exercise) and weight gain (it must work harder to pump blood through the arteries).

When the heart works harder, the coronary arteries dilate in order to make sure the heart has enough oxygen. Atherosclerosis, or a narrowing and "hardening" of the coronary arteries resulting from fatty deposits called plaque, reduces blood flow to the heart, causing injury to the heart muscle — a heart attack. If the reduction in blood flow is only temporary, there is no permanent damage, but the person may feel chest pain (angina).

Heart disease is more prevalent in the United States than in most other parts of the world; researchers blame our eating habits, excess weight, and sedentary lifestyle as leading causes. Poor methods of dealing with stress can also be an important factor. It is natural for the heart to work harder during stress — the "fight or flight" response that is built into our bodies to help us survive life-threatening situations. But when the "threat" is imagined, and the hormones (such as

adrenaline) and fats that have been mobilized for action are not used up, they continue circulating in the bloodstream, creating increased turbulence, which, along with the accelerated heart rate, increases the tension in the walls of the arteries — especially the coronary arteries. These may damage the lining of the arteries, which thickens as it heals, setting the stage for a possible blockage.

It is commonly thought that more men suffer from heart disease than women; this is true only until women reach menopause, when the odds of developing heart disease become the same for women as for men. It is thought that estrogen may protect women's hearts prior to menopause, when estrogen levels naturally begin to fall. Women with careers who also have the responsibilities of children and housework are particularly vulnerable to the harmful results of increased stress, including heart disease.

• *H*ow Yoga Can Help •

There are several risk factors that influence how likely you are to develop heart disease. Some, like heredity, you can't do anything about. But many, such as weight, smoking, exercise, diabetes, high cholesterol, high blood pressure, and how you respond to stress, can be changed. Yoga promotes the healthy lifestyle changes that will reduce your risk of developing heart disease — or help you get rid of it.

Research has shown that regular exercise reduces the likelihood of a heart attack by keeping the arteries from becoming clogged. Exercise also can reverse blockages if aerobic, strength, and flexibility training are combined in a balanced program. Exercise also seems to help people reduce other risk factors by helping to control weight, improving the body's ability to use insulin, conditioning the heart muscle, increasing levels of "good" HDL cholesterol, moderating stress, and lowering blood pressure. An exercise program enhances self-image and builds a sense of control over your health; this often inspires other positive lifestyle changes, such as eating a more healthful diet or stopping smoking.

If you are recovering from a heart attack, you may have the added stresses of depression, loss of self-esteem, fear of exerting yourself, and difficulty adjusting to new habits. Yoga exercise, breathing, and meditation will help by stimulating the release of chemicals in your brain that increase feelings of well-being and ease depression; increasing your strength and stamina so you feel better about yourself; and teaching you coping skills that will help you reduce stressful responses to life.

Recent studies have shown that including Yoga with other lifestyle changes can prevent or even correct heart problems, including atherosclerosis. Yoga has been recognized for some time as being effective in reducing high blood pressure, particularly the diastolic (lower) number, which is the most crucial. By integrating Yoga exercise, breathing, and meditation techniques into your day, you can make these important lifestyle changes. Yoga practice can make a real difference in the health of your heart by strengthening your nervous system, teaching you how to relax mentally and physically, and showing you how to better manage stress reactions.

Common stress reactions include muscle tension (most commonly in the face, stomach, neck, shoulders, and breath), rapid heart rate, constricted breathing, and anxiety. The fastest and most effective way to reduce reaction to stress is to change your breath, and an immediate way to improve your breathing is to improve your posture. In Yoga, you learn to strengthen your back and stomach muscles so that you can sit and stand straighter; this releases pressure on your heart and lungs and allows you to breathe easier.

Yoga breathing exercises teach you how to breathe more deeply and rhythmically; this has many effects, both physiological and mental. Physiologically, you will strengthen your respiratory muscles and develop a more efficient exchange of gases. Breathing exercises result in greater oxygenation of the blood. Mentally, you will notice more concentration, willpower, and steadiness.

Yoga exercise improves the health of the entire circulatory system, beginning with the production of blood, which takes place in the marrow of the long bones in the thighs, among other locations. Improving circulation in the legs by means of daily Yoga stretching exercises helps to rejuvenate the blood. Yoga exercises stretch the body's major blood vessels, keeping them free-flowing and elastic. Yoga oxygenates the blood and pushes fresh nutrients to all peripheral vessels and capillaries. Improved circulation means that your brain will receive more oxygen, improving alertness, memory, and mood; vital organs receive a steady supply of the nutrients they need for optimal functioning, and waste products are efficiently carried away and excreted.

Yoga relaxation training teaches you how to relax at will, allowing your body to release muscle tension almost as soon as it occurs. Meditation training shows you how to access your inner source of strength and personal power, creating a support system that builds confidence and self-esteem, fosters present-moment awareness, and increases self-awareness.

The choice to practice Yoga will protect your heart as it contributes to greater general health and well-being.

• Special Concerns •

Always consult your physician before beginning any new exercise program. Many of the techniques described in this chapter can be done in chairs if your doctor advises you to begin more slowly. See individual technique instructions for variations. The recommended floor exercises (Hands and Knees Stretch, Knee Squeeze, Pelvic Twist, Cobra Pose, and Tortoise Stretch) can also be done in bed.

Things You Can Do Throughout the Day

"Take a breather": Practice stress-coping techniques such as the Complete Breath to reduce your recovery time from harmful stress responses. If you are sitting down most of the day, get up every hour or two and do some simple stretches such as Full Bends, Alternate Triangle, Windmill, and Spine Twist. See the technique instructions below for suggestions on how to adapt some of the exercises so you can practice them sitting in a chair.

Learn to recognize the types of situations that commonly "set you off" and develop a substitute response to them. When you find yourself in a stressful situation, such as being stuck in slow-moving traffic, practice relaxation responses such as the Belly Breath, and some easy tension-reducing exercises such as Shoulder Roll, Neck Stretch, and Standing Twist. Without closing your eyes, isolate and relax the muscles in your forehead, eyes, jaw, shoulders, and stomach. Remember that it is not the source of stress itself that causes the harm to your body, but your response to it.

Practice flexibility: See if you can go for a whole day — or even just a whole hour — saying "okay" to anything that is put in front of you (barring anything destructive or violent, of course). If you have perfectionistic tendencies, this exercise may be a real challenge for you. But if you practice regularly, you will find a restful feeling taking the place of constant anxiety throughout your day.

Use the "I Love You" meditation technique (pp. 28-29) to comfort your mind and body.

Dietary Suggestions

If you are at high risk for heart disease, it goes without saying that you must start immediately to change your diet to one that is heart-healthy. Reduce fats — especially polysaturated fats — drastically, and eat meals high in the stress-fighting nutrients: protein, calcium, and vitamins C and B-complex. If you are trying to lose weight, avoid "fad" diets; consult a reputable nutritionist or a good book for a balanced program that keeps you strong while you lose weight (see Appendix B, Further Reading).

Daily Routine for Heart Disease

Start with the basic routine described in Chapter 1, then incorporate the special exercises in this chapter. These exercises have been chosen because they improve circulation through compression, improve breathing by expanding the chest wall, function as stress-coping techniques that can be done throughout the day, increase elasticity in the blood vessel walls, and increase awareness of muscle tension so that it can be relaxed.

If you don't have time to do a full routine, do at least three warmup exercises and three of the exercises described below, and always do at least a few minutes of meditation. Best results will be obtained if you practice every day.

Here is a list of the full sequence of techniques (including the basic routine):

Complete Breath, p. 26
Warmups, pp. 16-20
Dancer Pose, p. 104
Thigh Stretch, p. 105
Standing Sun Pose, p. 21
Baby Pose, p. 24
Camel Pose, p. 105
Frog Pose, p. 105
Hands and Knees Stretch, p. 106
Spine Twist, pp. 106-107 (This exercise can also be done in a chair. See below.)
Seated Sun Pose, p. 22
Tortoise Stretch, p. 23
Knee Squeeze, p. 107 (This exercise can also be done in a chair. See below.)
Pelvic Twist, p. 108
Cobra Pose, p. 108
Relaxation and Meditation, pp. 26-27

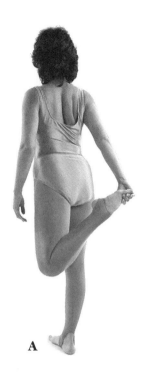

A

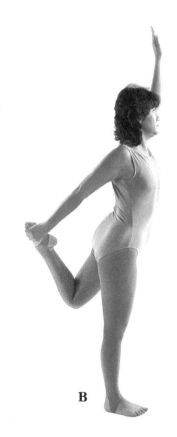

B

Dancer Pose.   *Strengthens the lower back; limbers and strengthens the hips and thighs; improves mental poise; improves posture, balance, and concentration; strengthens ankles; relieves upper back tension.* Throughout the exercise, steady yourself by fixing your gaze on one spot on the wall in front of you. From a standing rest position, bend your right knee and grasp your right foot in back with your left hand (**A**). Check to be sure your stomach muscles are relaxed and your breathing steady. Slowly move into the completed Dancer Pose by raising your right arm straight up toward the ceiling so it is next to your ear and pulling your right leg up and back as far as possible without strain (**B**). Don't lean forward, and keep your supporting leg straight. Relax your stomach, breathe normally, and keep your gaze fixed on one spot. Hold for a count of three, then carefully return to the beginning position. [3 times each side.]

For more of a challenge: add the **Dancer Pose Extension**. Try this extension after you have become proficient in the Dancer Pose. From the Dancer position after your 3-count hold as described above, maintain your gaze and, still breathing normally, slowly lower your body into the extended position (**C**). In addition to the benefits of the Dancer Pose, this variation stretches the back of the legs and increases strength and stamina. Keep your right leg as far up and back as possible. Your right arm extends straight ahead. Your left (supporting) leg remains straight. Stare at one spot for balance and hold for a count of three. Don't strain. Come back to a standing rest position.

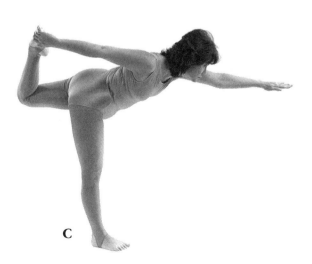

C

Thigh Stretch. *Stretches all muscles of the legs and hips; improves respiration; increases circulation.* Stand with feet apart a comfortable distance and swivel to face left. Bend forward and place your hands on either side of your left foot. Bend your left leg, lower your hips, breathe in, arch your back and look up (**A**). Hold for a count of three. Now breathe out and straighten your legs, keeping the toes of your left foot pointed and tucking your head in toward your left leg (**B**). Hold for a count of three. [3 each side]

Camel Pose. *Limbers entire spine; improves circulation and respiration; stretches and strengthens thighs and knees; improves functioning of thyroid; strengthens heart.* Kneel with legs slightly separated. The first two movements in this exercise help to prepare the spine for an intense stretch: Carefully bend back and grasp your left heel with your left hand. Push your hips forward slightly (**C**). Repeat on the right side. Now bend backward and grasp one heel with each hand. Push your hips forward as far as possible and let your head relax back (**D**) (unless you have neck problems, in which case do not let your head drop backward). Hold for a count of three, breathing normally. As you get stronger, you can repeat if you wish. Release and rest briefly in the Baby Pose. [1 repetition]

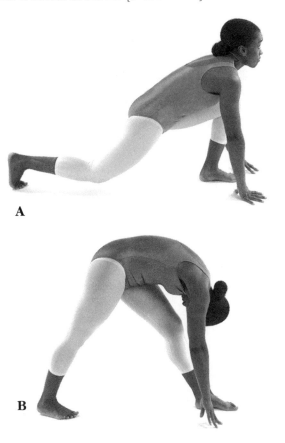

A

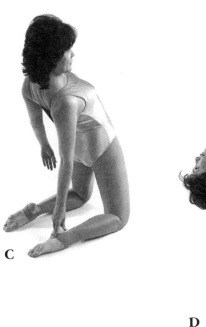

C

B

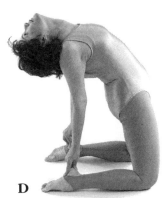

D

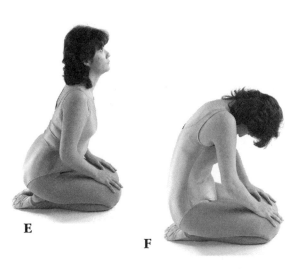

E

F

Frog Pose. *Limbers rib cage and lower spine; improves respiration and posture.* Sit on your feet with knees together (if this position is uncomfortable, the exercise can be done sitting in a chair with feet flat on the floor). Place your hands on your knees. Breathe in deeply as you arch your back and look up, stretching your throat and leaning forward slightly (**E**). Hold for a count of three. Breathe out as you bend the opposite way, rounding your back and tucking your chin into your chest (**F**). Hold for a count of three. [3 repetitions]

Hands and Knees Stretch. *Limbers lower back; stretches chest muscles; loosens hip and knee joints; improves respiration.* Sitting on your feet on the floor, breathe out through your nose. Breathe in as you come forward on all fours, then lower your hips, arch your back and look up, keeping your arms stiff (**A**). Breathe out and sit back, bending forward with arms stretched out in front (**B**), then breathe in back to position (**A**). [3 repetitions]

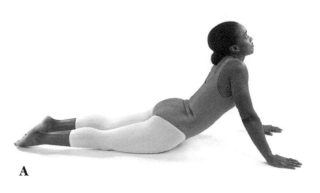

A

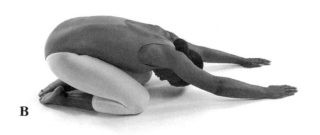

B

Spine Twist. *Improves digestion; limbers and tones entire spine; strengthens and limbers rib cage; relieves chronic constipation; helps relieve bladder, urinary tract, and prostate problems; strengthens heart.* Bend both knees. Rest your right leg on the floor, and lift your left leg over the right knee; the left foot should be flat (**C**). Sit up very straight, reach your right arm across your left knee, push the knee as far right as it will go, and grasp your left ankle; this locks the lower back into position (**D**). (Alternatively, if you are unable to reach your left ankle, grasp your right knee instead. You can also simply hook your right arm over your left knee and straighten the leg, as in **F**.) Now place your left arm behind you, straighten it and point the fingers in toward the base of your spine. Look forward, breathe in, then breathe out and twist toward the left as far as possible. Look far to the left with your eyes and stare at one spot (**E**). Hold for a count of three, breathing gently, and do not blink. As you get stronger, you can increase the holding time. Then release and slowly come forward. [3 times each direction]

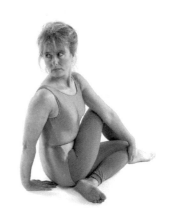

E

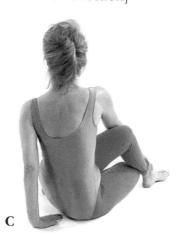

C

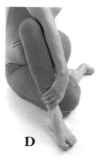

D

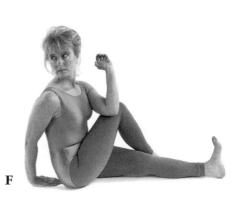

F

Chair variation: Seated Twist. Sit up straight in your chair, with feet flat on the floor. Place your right hand on the outside of your left knee. Place your left arm across the back of the chair, or inside the back of the chair, or in any comfortable position that pulls the left arm back slightly. Grasp the chair back or seat firmly. Sit up straight, and breathe in completely. Breathe out as you slowly turn toward the left as far as you can (**A**). Pull with your right hand to get the greatest stretch. Turn your head as far toward the left as you can, and look to the left with your eyes. Hold for a count of three. Now breathe in as you slowly return to face front. Relax. Repeat on the other side. [3 times each direction]

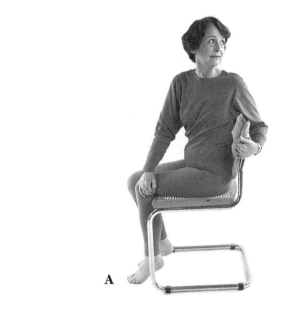

A

Knee Squeeze. *Improves digestion; limbers and relaxes lower back and hips; improves circulation in pelvic region; removes poisons from the body.* Lie on your back with arms over your head on the floor. Breathe out completely. Keeping your right knee straight, breathe in, bend your left knee, and lift your head, wrapping your arms around the knee. Hold your breath in and squeeze your knee to your chest (**B**). Hold for a count of three, then release, breathe out, and lower the leg and arms back to the starting position. [3 times each side, alternating]

After 3 repetitions on each side, do the same exercise lifting both legs at once (**C**). [3 repetitions]

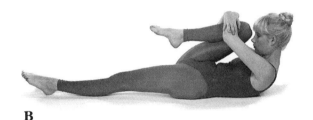

B

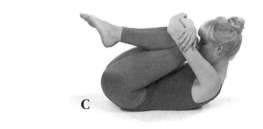

C

Chair variation: Seated Knee Squeeze. Sit up straight away from the back of your chair with your arms at your sides. Start by slowly breathing out as much air as possible. Now breathe in, lift your right knee up high, and squeeze it to your chest with both hands. Bend your forehead to your knee and hold for a count of three (**D**). As you slowly breathe out, relax your arms and lower your leg to the floor. [3 times each side]

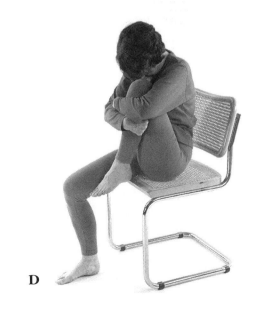

D

Pelvic Twist. *Compresses internal organs, stimulating circulation and metabolism; reduces waistline; strengthens lower back and legs.* Lie on your back with your arms outstretched, palms down. Bend your knees and bring them up toward your chest (**A**). This is your starting position. Breathe in as you slowly swing your legs toward the left as far as possible (keep knees bent). Hold for a count of three, then breathe out as you lift your legs back to your starting position. Breathe out and swing them to the opposite side. Hold for a count of three. [3 on each side, alternating]

After you've practiced this for several weeks, and if you have no back or neck problems, try a more difficult variation: when you swing your legs to the side, straighten them as they reach the ground (**B**), then bend them as they come back up to your starting position. The breathing pattern is the same. [3 each side, alternating]

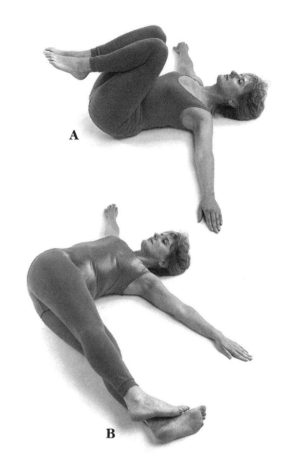

Cobra Pose. *Improves functioning of digestive, respiratory, and reproductive systems; limbers and strengthens entire spine; strengthens eyesight; equalizes two sides of body; improves complexion.* Lie on your stomach with legs together (those with occasional lower back trouble should separate the legs at first). Place your forehead on the floor and your palms down next to your armpits close to your body so your elbows point back and up, not out to the sides (**C**). Breathe out completely, then start to breathe in as you curl first your head and eyes back as far as they will go, then your chest, and then your stomach (**D**). Keep your hipbones on the floor — this is not a push-up — and your arms slightly bent (unless you are extremely limber). Use your back muscles more than your arms. Hold for a count of three at the top with your breath in and eyes looking up through your forehead. Do not blink. Then start to breathe out and curl forward slowly, in reverse: your stomach curls down first, then your chest, and finally your head and eyes. Your eyes are the first part of your body to curl up and the last to curl down. [3 repetitions]

Caution: This is a very powerful exercise and should not be done if you have had recent surgery or by women during the menstrual period, as it encourages blood flow.

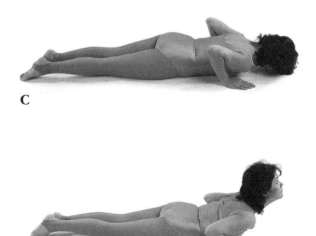

Type A's, Move Over

Studies show that negative emotions such as anger, depression, and anxiety are major factors in the development of heart disease. Negative emotions tax the immune system as well, increasing susceptibility to disease. A recent study found that the "Type A" personality — characterized by the driven, perfectionistic qualities previously thought to make a person most susceptible to heart disease — is only a factor if the person also has a high degree of hostility. The new theory has been dubbed "Type H."

If this sounds like you, you may find that a regular Yoga program, combined with professional counseling and medical care, can help you change the way you react to the world around you. Often hostility and other negative reactions such as fear, anger, and depression are simply habits formed from long years of responding to life's crises in a certain way. These behaviors can be changed, and Yoga can provide the inner strength to support such changes.

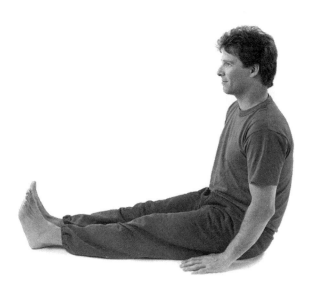

Infertility
Chapter 12

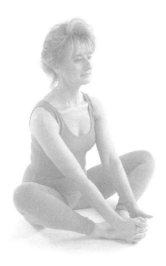

Couples who seem to be unable to conceive often describe their feelings as an "emotional roller-coaster" alternating between hope and despair. Infertility usually precipitates a series of crises — which means never-ending stress: there is the monthly anxiety of new tests and treatments, and the disappointment when conception fails yet again. Couples face overwhelming physical, financial, and emotional pressures that seem to take over their lives. Their usual coping skills may not work in the face of repeated failure and feelings of helplessness.

At least 15 percent of Americans experience infertility or impotence, and there has been a dramatic rise in numbers in the past 30 years. Lifestyle changes, pollution, increased use of chemicals in food and the environment — there are many theories about why these problems have increased. I believe that infertility problems are seldom due entirely to organic causes, but are clearly related to stress. There are heavy demands on both men and women in our society today from all sides; the pressure to produce in the working world cannot help but affect biological systems as well.

A person can only produce so much, and the production of beautiful children requires a tremendous amount of effort in the emotional nature. It is unseen but very powerful.

When men and women are both under pressure to produce at work, their energy is diverted, leaving little to produce a child. It is necessary for you to put energy back into the emotional and physical systems to take care of this extra demand on your body and emotions.

This can be seen so clearly in the phenomenon, so common, of a couple giving up on having a child and adopting one — and then almost immediately getting pregnant! It's very possible that the energy of the parents, instead of being totally directed toward work, was redirected toward the adopted child, and that extra attention and energy allowed the birth of another child. Children are born not just because of physical conception but because of other, more subtle, factors which can be encouraged.

• *H*ow Yoga Can Help •

Both men and women in this country are brought up to give and give and give. When you sacrifice yourself completely to your job or to your family, you get a large measure of approval, no matter what the cost. Yoga says that you have to "put some water back into the well" in order to have something to give. You must learn how to replace the vital attention and needs of the body and mind. This can be done easily with a simple 30-minute routine of exercise, breathing, and meditation, and careful attention to nutrition. Among other benefits, Yoga exercises bring the systems of your body into perfect balance — including the reproductive system in both men and women. Compression poses are especially beneficial because they stimulate the body's glandular system and help regulate metabolism. Yoga exercises practiced every day replenish and rebalance the physical and emotional systems that are depleted by the everyday stresses that lie so heavy on our lives.

Relaxation and meditation techniques are universally recommended for coping with stress. In guided relaxation sessions, you learn how to relax every muscle and bone in your body — even those systems, like your heartbeat and breath, which are automatic — so your body and mind get a complete rest. In meditation training, you learn how to let go of anxious thoughts about the future or despairing thoughts about the past and, instead, rest in the present moment. Daily practice of Yoga builds a support system of confidence and strength from within that stays with you throughout the day.

• Things You Can Do Throughout the Day •

Learn the "I Love You" meditation technique (pp. 28-29) and remember how you feel when you are doing it; recalling this feeling will reinforce self-confidence and self-acceptance throughout the day.

Use the Complete Breath (p. 26) to reduce harmful stress reactions or to lift depression.

Practice the Laughasan exercise (p. 117) several times a day, and set aside some time to play every day.

Welcome your child in your meditation. Fantasize about your baby every day; see every detail in your mind.

• Dietary Suggestions •

Eat a balanced, anti-stress diet rich in low-fat protein, complex carbohydrates, and fresh fruits and vegetables. Avoid alcohol, excessive caffeine, artificial foods and chemicals, and overly processed foods.

• Daily Routine for Infertility •

Start with the basic routine described in Chapter 1, then incorporate the special exercises in this chapter. These exercises have been chosen because they build emotional stability, compress the glands and organs to stimulate the hormonal system and balance metabolism, improve functioning of the reproductive system, enhance self-esteem, and increase relaxation. Compression poses are especially helpful in cases of impotency.

If you don't have time to do a full routine, do at least three warmup exercises and three of the exercises described below, and always do the full relaxation procedure and at least a few minutes of meditation. Best results will be gained from practicing whatever techniques you choose once in every 24-hour period.

Here is a list of the full sequence of techniques (including the basic routine):

Complete Breath, p. 26
Warmups, pp. 16-20
Standing Knee Squeeze, p. 112
Standing Sun Pose, p. 21
Cobra V-Raise, p. 112
Baby Pose, p. 24
Thigh Stretch, p. 112
Hero Variation, p. 113
Seated Sun Pose, p. 22
Tortoise Stretch, p. 23
Pigeon Pose, p. 113
Diamond Pose, p. 114
Knee Squeeze, p. 114
Shoulder Stand, p. 115
Easy Bridge, p. 116
Cobra Pose, p. 116
Swan Dive, p. 117
Relaxation and Meditation, pp. 26-27
Laughasan, p. 117

Standing Knee Squeeze. *Improves digestion and balance, strengthens legs and feet, improves circulation in upper body, helps relieve stiffness in hips and knees.* Stand with feet together next to a chair, barre, or other sturdy support. Holding on with your right hand, breathe out completely. Then breathe in as you lift your left leg, bending the knee and wrapping your left arm (not just your hand) around the knee. Hold your breath in as you squeeze the knee toward your chest and bend your forehead down toward your knee (**A**). Hold for a count of three. Release and lower the leg. When you are comfortable with this exercise, and if your balance is good, grasp your upraised knee with both arms for a more intense compression (**B**). [3 times on each side]

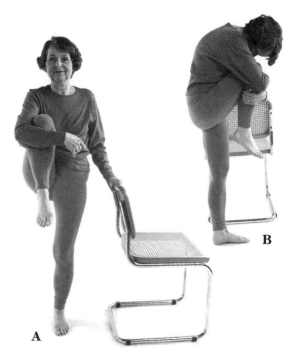

A

B

Thigh Stretch. *Stretches all muscles of the legs and hips; improves respiration; increases circulation.* Stand with feet apart a comfortable distance and swivel to face left. Bend forward and place your hands on either side of your left foot. Bend your left leg, lower your hips, breathe in, arch your back and look up (**E**). Hold for a count of three. Now breathe out and straighten your legs, keeping the toes of your left foot pointed and tucking your head in toward your left leg (**F**). Hold for a count of three. [3 each side]

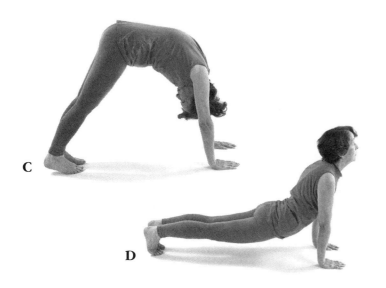

C

D

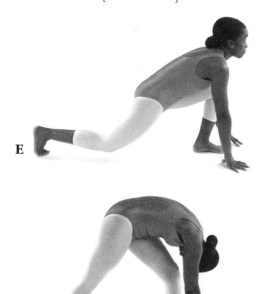

E

F

Cobra V-Raise. *Strengthens legs, back, shoulders, and rib cage; strengthens heart; improves functioning of the organs in the pelvic region; reduces body fat.* Walk your hands forward on the floor, keeping your heels down as far as possible, until your hands are about 4 to 5 feet in front of you. Tuck your chin into your chest and breathe out. This is the "V" position (**C**). Now, keeping your arms straight, breathe in and slowly lower your body, arching your back and looking up and back (**D**) (the "cobra" position). Hold for a count of three. Push back slowly into the V position, breathing out and tucking your chin into your chest. Hold for a count of three. [3 repetitions]

Hero Variation.   *Stretches rib cage; improves respiration; limbers upper back and shoulders.* In a kneeling position, clasp your hands in back and straighten your arms (**A**). Breathe in completely. Breathe out and bend forward, keeping your arms straight and pulled away from your body as much as possible (**B**). Hold for a count of three. Breathe in and come back up. [3 repetitions]

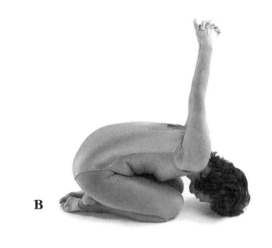
B

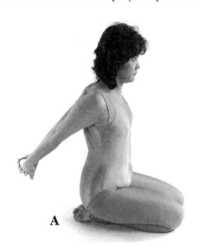
A

Pigeon Pose & Hold.   *Stretches, strengthens, and tones spinal column, hip joints, and groin muscles; stimulates metabolic system; improves breathing.* From a kneeling position, slide your left leg straight back and sit on your right heel. Bend forward and rest your chest on your right thigh, and place your hands palms down on either side of your knee. Place your forehead on the floor and relax completely (**C**). Breathe out. Breathe in as you slowly curl your eyes, head, and chest up and back as far as you can comfortably (**D**). Hold for a count of three, looking up. Slowly breathe out as you curl down, bringing your chest down first, then your head and eyes. [3 repetitions]

After your third repetition, make fists and push your upper body up. Keep your legs and hips relaxed and your neck straight. Look at one spot on the floor. Tuck your left toes under (**E**). Hold for several seconds, breathing normally. Then switch sides: Push yourself up on all fours, stretching your right leg back straight and bringing your left leg forward. Repeat the entire sequence.

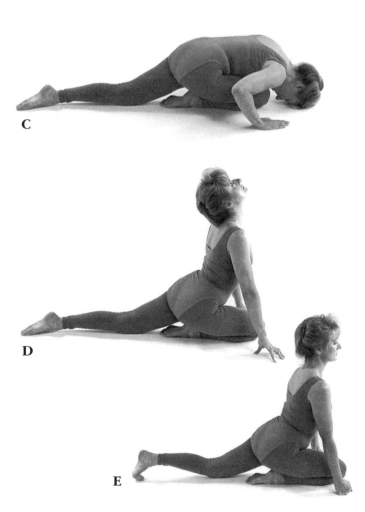
C

D

E

Diamond Pose. *Limbers lower back, hips and groin muscles; releases back tension.* Sit straight with knees bent and the soles of your feet touching. Grasp your ankles with both hands and rest your elbows on or above your thighs. Breathe in completely, then breathe out as you lean forward slightly and press down on your thighs with your arms. Hold for a count of three. Release and repeat twice more. Now lace your fingers around your toes, breathe in, and straighten your spine (**A**). Breathe out as you bend forward, letting your elbows fall outside your legs this time (**B**). Hold for a count of three, then breathe in and come back up. [3 repetitions]

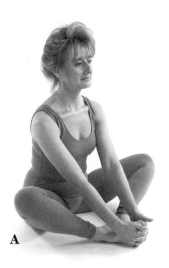

A

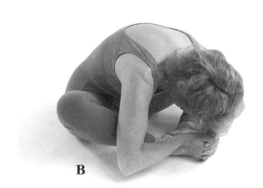

B

Knee Squeeze. *Improves digestion; limbers and relaxes lower back and hips; improves circulation in pelvic region; removes poisons from the body.* Lie on your back with arms over your head on the floor. Breathe out completely. Keeping your right knee straight, breathe in, bend your left knee, and lift your head, wrapping your arms around the knee. Hold your breath in and squeeze your knee to your chest (**C**). Hold for a count of three, then release, breathe out, and lower the leg and arms back to the starting position. [3 times each side, alternating]

After 3 repetitions on each side, do the same exercise lifting both legs at once (**D**). [3 repetitions]

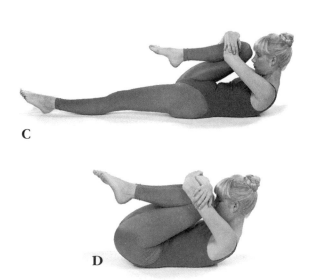

C

D

Shoulder Stand. *Stimulates thyroid and parathyroid; enhances function of all vital organs; relieves tension on heart and lungs; relaxes nervous system; removes fatigue.* If you have a disk problem in your neck, do not do this exercise; substitute the Easy Bridge (p. 116) instead. Start by sitting with knees drawn up to chest and arms wrapped around knees (**A**). Gently roll back and forth a few times (**B**) to make sure that the spine is in place with no pinched nerves or strained muscles. Then roll back, keeping knees to forehead, and immediately support your lower back with your hands and keep your knees bent and your body in the rounded position (**C**). Hold this position until you feel steady, then slowly straighten your legs toward the ceiling (**D**). If your legs appear to be more at a 45° angle, move your hands down your back toward the floor, push gently, and tuck your chin into your chest; your legs should straighten a bit more. Fix your gaze on the ceiling in the space between your big toes. Relax your breath. Hold for a count of three. As you get stronger, you can increase the hold to one-half minute, up to a full minute (do not exceed one minute). Women should not do this exercise during the menstrual period.

Come out of the pose by bending your knees and bringing them to your forehead. Cross your ankles (**E**) and slowly roll forward, rounding your back, until you come all the way up to a seated position. Bend forward for a few seconds to be sure the blood doesn't drain from your head too fast. [1 repetition]

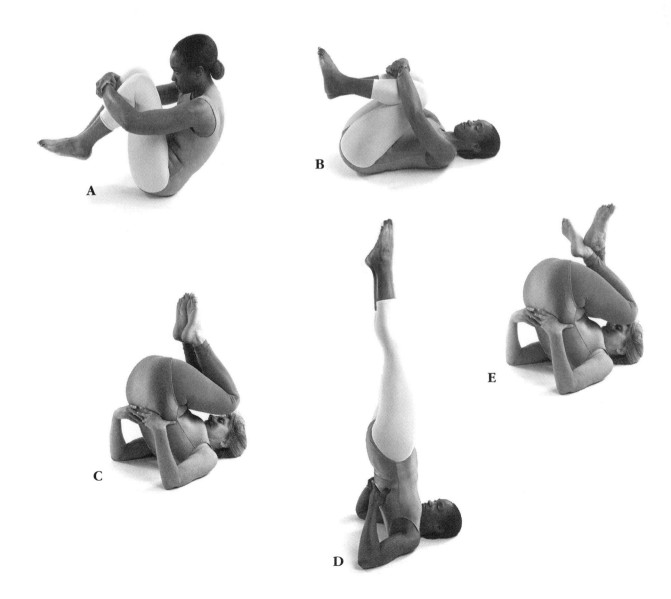

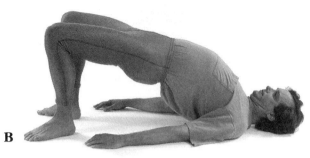

A

B

Easy Bridge. *Improves functioning of thyroid; eases back pain and fatigue; increases circulation to head; helps relieve bedsores.* Lying on your back, bend your knees and bring your feet as close to your hips as possible. Separate your feet several inches. Place your arms palms down at your sides. Relax your neck and upper back, breathe out completely, pushing your waist to the floor slightly, then breathe in and raise your hips, curling up just to your waist (**A**) (your back will be rounded and your chin tucked toward your chest). Hold for a count of three, then breathe out and lower. Next, breathe in and lift your hips as high as you can without strain, keeping your shoulders on the floor and arching your back (**B**). Your chin will be tucked into your chest. Hold for a count of three, then slowly lower and breathe out. As you become more limber, you can hold onto your ankles for a greater stretch. [3 repetitions each variation]

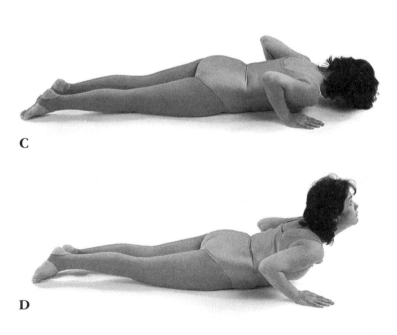

C

D

Cobra Pose. *Improves functioning of digestive, respiratory, and reproductive systems; limbers and strengthens entire spine; strengthens eyesight; equalizes two sides of body; improves complexion.* Lie on your stomach with legs together (those with occasional lower back trouble should separate the legs at first). Place your forehead on the floor and your palms down next to your armpits close to your body so your elbows point back and up, not out to the sides (**C**). Breathe out completely, then start to breathe in as you curl first your head and eyes back as far as they will go, then your chest, and then your stomach (**D**). Keep your hipbones on the floor — this is not a push-up — and your arms slightly bent (unless you are extremely limber). Use your back muscles more than your arms. Hold for a count of three at the top with your breath in and eyes looking up through your forehead. Do not blink. Then start to breathe out and curl forward slowly, in reverse: your stomach curls down first, then your chest, and finally your head and eyes. Your eyes are the first part of your body to curl up and the last to curl down. [3 repetitions]

Caution: This is a very powerful exercise and should not be done if you have had recent surgery or by women during the menstrual period, as it encourages blood flow.

Swan Dive.   *Strengthens back, leg, and shoulder muscles; massages internal organs; improves circulation to the spine and brain.* Lie on your stomach with your legs together, your arms stretched out to the sides, and your forehead on the floor. Breathe out. Breathe in as you lift arms, legs, and head, looking up through your forehead (**A**). Hold for a count of three. Breathe out and relax back to the starting position. [3 repetitions]

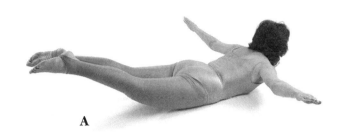

A

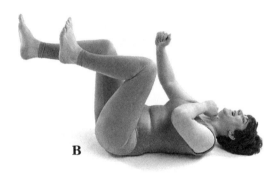

B

Laughasan.   *Relieves muscle tension in the entire body; activates the immune system and releases endorphins.* Lie on your back and start pumping your legs as if you were riding a bicycle. Move your arms, too, and start to laugh. Pump your arms and legs as vigorously as you can and laugh out loud for at least 30 seconds (**B**).

Making Time for Yourself

Often the hardest task for new students of Yoga is to make the commitment to practice every day. If you are someone who works hard, plays hard, and has an active social life, there may be many days when you find yourself on the go from early morning until late at night. Setting aside 30 minutes or so for Yoga may be difficult at first, but you will reap the rewards over time as you begin to notice a greater sense of well-being. Many people like to do their Yoga routine in the morning, because they feel less distracted at that time. If you don't enjoy the early morning hours, you may wish to practice in the late afternoon, after work. If so, be sure to shower beforehand to relax your body and to symbolically wash away the problems of the day. Practicing in the late evening is another possibility, although you may be tired by then and unable to concentrate the way you'd like. Also, some people find that exercising in the late evening keeps them awake because of the stimulating effect of the exercises.

If none of these times suits your schedule, you can split up the routine: exercise in the morning to add extra energy to your day, and do the breathing and meditation in the afternoon or evening when you will welcome the relaxing effects. Remember, the most important point is to practice every day, no matter what time of day you choose.

Insomnia
Chapter 13

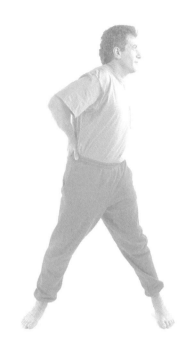

Difficulty in falling or staying asleep can hinder all aspects of life. People with sleep problems often feel irritable, tense, helpless, and depressed. A sleep disturbance can develop from a minor annoyance to a debilitating and self-perpetuating cycle if not treated. Sleep loss accumulates. A person with a big sleep debt is slower to recover from stress and is much more vulnerable to infections and other illnesses and to the effects of alcohol.

Sleep is necessary for the body's restorative functions; Shakespeare referred to "Sleep that knits up the ravell'd sleave of care." In sleep, the body and brain seem to be doing less; but in fact they are very active in a different way, rebuilding muscle tissue and performing other necessary functions.

Insomnia often appears when your lifestyle or environment are disrupted, or when you feel especially worried about work or personal problems. The drive to succeed at a career, to maintain a happy family structure, and to build a satisfying social life creates pressures to rest less and produce more. Insomnia may result from depression, anxiety, or other psychological problems, or from medical or behavioral causes, such as a hormonal upset, a painful situation or illness, a reaction to medication, an allergy, your diet, smoking, or drinking too much alcohol before going to bed.

Insomnia afflicts people of all ages and backgrounds but is more prevalent among women and people who are single. About 80 million Americans say they have trouble sleeping, but only a small percentage seek a doctor's advice for the problem. Women seek help for their insomnia more often than men do, and women are much more likely to have sleeping pills prescribed for them. Daytime sleepiness, surprisingly, seems to be more prevalent than the inability to sleep at night. In one survey, more than a third of persons over the age of 50 said they suffered from insomnia, indicating that sleep disturbances become more likely with age.

Many people automatically reach for sleeping pills when they have trouble sleeping. Unfortunately, this usually does more harm than good: pills often have side effects, they rarely address the cause of the sleep problem, they can lead to dependency, and they can even make the insomnia worse. Moreover, they discourage trying other ways to get enough rest. Using alcohol to sleep doesn't work either because it prevents the deep sleep that is the most restorative stage of sleep.

• *H*ow Yoga Can Help •

If you suffer from insomnia, whether often or occasionally, Yoga can help. Through relaxing physical exercise, breathing techniques, and complete relaxation, you can promote more regular and restful sleeping patterns without resorting to drugs. Through Yoga practice, you can rest the mind by learning to stop continual thought.

If you have difficulty getting to sleep, and if your doctor has ruled out medical causes, try the deep relaxation and meditation (see Chapter 1) in a lying-down position 30 minutes before bed. This procedure works by relaxing each part of your body and then stopping mental conversation for a few minutes, relieving the mind of the constant barrage of thoughts, memories, anxieties, and reactions that keep you awake. Most anxious thoughts have to do with either the past or the future; meditation teaches you how to be more aware in the present moment, which produces a deep rest. Keeping our relaxation and meditation tape next to your bed with earphones to be used in the night as needed is especially helpful (see Resources).

If you awaken during the night, practice the Complete Breath (Chapter 1) while lying on your back. By focusing on the sound and rhythm of the breath, it will relax your mind and body, and it will lead you back to sleep before you know it. During the day, this breathing exercise can be practiced anytime to interrupt racing thoughts and give yourself a break from stress. Taking a warm shower or bath as soon as you come home from work, moreover, will make your evening more relaxing by removing the stresses of the day.

A daily routine of Yoga exercises can also minimize other symptoms that may cause insomnia. Physical exercises that stretch and relax the muscles help reduce fatigue and stress, while keeping your physical systems at optimum health. Some people experience a stimulating effect when they do the exercises in the late evening; if this is the case for you, do your exercises in the morning or afternoon instead.

Always do a meditation session after your Yoga exercises. Meditation will help train your mind and body to stop thinking and stop moving. It trains you to turn inward to a peaceful silence which encourages sleep. Daily practice of 15 to 30 minutes will give you the best results. Because the complete relaxation process of beginning meditation is so similar to preparation for sleep, most people go through a stage in beginning practice when they actually fall asleep in meditation. This kind of sleep, however, is very different because it is much deeper and more restful.

• *T*hings You Can Do Throughout the Day •

Practice present-moment awareness. What is happening right now? What am I doing now? What am I feeling now? Use Yoga breathing techniques to help you focus on the present. Every time you notice yourself with anxious or fearful thoughts, do a few Complete Breath exercises and concentrate only on the sound of the breath.

Recognize physical tension and relax it. Regularly check your jaw, forehead, shoulders, back, and stomach. If your joints and muscles feel tight, do some loosening exercises such as the Shoulder Roll, Full Bend, Elbow Twist, and Standing Reach (see Chapter 1).

• Dietary Suggestions •

Many sources recommend avoiding caffeinated beverages for at least six hours before bedtime, and avoiding alcohol or a heavy meal right before bed (but it is a good idea to get plenty of water during the day). If you want a snack before bed, eat a complex carbohydrate such as bread or pasta; avoid sugary, high-fat, or high-protein foods.

• Daily Routine for Insomnia •

Start with the basic routine described in Chapter 1, then incorporate the special exercises in this chapter. These exercises have been chosen because they improve circulation, stretch and relax major muscle groups through the use of "whole body" exercises, oxygenate the blood, help you develop greater concentration and focus on the present moment, and improve respiration.

If you don't have time to do a full routine, do at least three warmup exercises and three of the exercises described below, and always do the full relaxation procedure and a few minutes of meditation. Best results will be obtained if you practice at least a few techniques every day without fail.

Here is a list of the full sequence of techniques (including the basic routine):

Complete Breath, p. 26
Warmups, pp. 16-20
Standing Knee Squeeze, p. 121
Twisting Triangle, p. 121
Windmill, p. 122
Dancer Pose, p. 122
Tree Pose, p. 123
Standing Sun Pose, p. 21
Baby Pose, p. 24
Seated Sun Pose, p. 22
Tortoise Stretch, p. 23
Cat Breath, p. 123
Alternate Toe Touch, p. 124
Shoulder Stand, p. 124
Easy Cobra, p. 125
Boat Pose, p. 125
Laughasan, p. 125
Relaxation and Meditation, pp. 26-27

The Power of Water

It is said that Yogis love water because it has no resistance. As such, water represents the ultimate adaptability to change. Using this idea, you can use water to change the way you feel. When you take a shower or bath, think of the water washing away bad moods, anxious thoughts, and other people's troubles — you'll be "starting fresh" in more ways than one. If you find yourself feeling upset at work, splash some water on your hands and face in the restroom and imagine the water helping you return to a calmer state of mind. And it's a good idea to always bathe before bed for a more restful sleep.

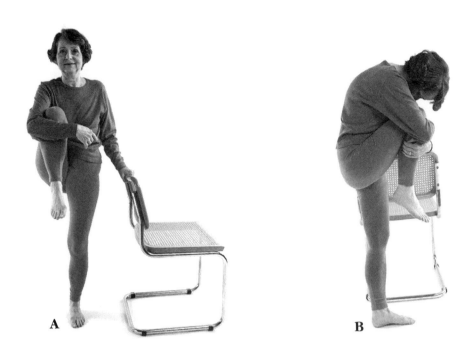

A   B

Standing Knee Squeeze. *Improves digestion and balance, strengthens legs and feet, improves circulation in upper body, helps relieve stiffness in hips and knees.* Stand with feet together next to a chair, barre, or other sturdy support. Holding on with your right hand, breathe out completely. Then breathe in as you lift your left leg, bending the knee and wrapping your left arm (not just your hand) around the knee. Hold your breath in as you squeeze the knee toward your chest and bend your forehead down toward your knee (**A**). Hold for a count of three. Release and lower the leg. When you are comfortable with this exercise, and if your balance is good, grasp your upraised knee with both arms for a more intense compression (**B**). [3 times on each side]

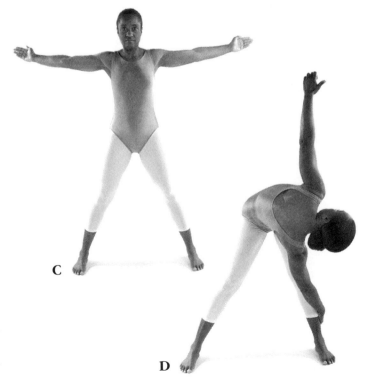

C

D

Twisting Triangle. *Increases flexibility and circulation in hips and lower back; strengthens hip joints and upper back; helps relieve depression.* Separate your feet as wide as you can comfortably (without losing your balance) and point your toes forward. Breathe in and raise your arms to the sides, parallel to the floor (**C**). Breathe out as you bend toward the left leg, grasp the outside of your left ankle (or calf) with your right hand, then turn your head so you are looking at your left hand, which should be pointed straight up, fingers curled and thumb toward you (**D**). Stare at your thumb. You can pull slightly with your right hand to increase the stretch. Keep both knees straight. Hold for a count of three, then breathe in and come back to your starting position, arms outstretched. [3 times each side, alternating]

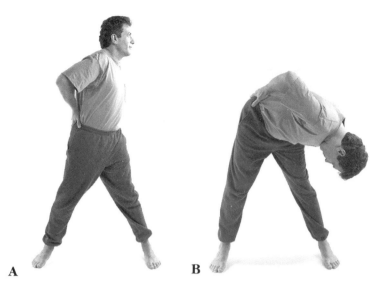

A　　　　B

Windmill. *Limbers and strengthens lower back, hip joints, and upper thigh; improves respiration; reduces waistline.* Stand with your feet as far apart as you can comfortably, toes pointed in. Place your hands on your lower back, thumbs over your hips and fingers supporting your lower back. Start by breathing in completely and turning toward the left (**A**). Breathe out as you bend your head toward your left leg (**B**) and continue moving over to your right leg. Now start to breathe in as you come back to a standing position and face front. Finish breathing in completely. Repeat twice more in the same direction. Your breathing pattern in this exercise follows the circular movements of your head: You are breathing out for two-thirds of the circle (from standing, over to the left leg, then to the right leg) and breathing in for the remaining third of the circle (as you stand up). [3 slow circles each direction]

Dancer Pose. *Strengthens the lower back; limbers and strengthens the hips and thighs; improves mental poise; improves posture, balance, and concentration; strengthens ankles; relieves upper back tension.* Throughout the exercise, steady yourself by fixing your gaze on one spot on the wall in front of you. From a standing rest position, bend your right knee and grasp your right foot in back with your left hand (**C**). Check to be sure your stomach muscles are relaxed and your breathing steady. Slowly move into the completed Dancer Pose by raising your right arm straight up toward the ceiling so it is next to your ear and pulling your right leg up and back as far as possible without strain (**D**). Don't lean forward, and keep your supporting leg straight. Relax your stomach, breathe normally, and keep your gaze fixed on one spot. Hold for a count of three, then carefully return to the beginning position. [3 times each side]

For more of a challenge: add the **Dancer Pose Extension**. Try this extension after you have become proficient in the Dancer Pose. From the Dancer position after your 3-count hold as described above, maintain your gaze and, still breathing normally, slowly lower your body into the extended position (**E**). In addition to the benefits of the Dancer Pose, this variation stretches the back of the legs and increases strength and stamina. Keep your right leg as far up and back as possible. Your right arm extends straight ahead. Your left (supporting) leg remains straight. Stare at one spot for balance and hold for a count of three. Don't strain. Come back to a standing rest position.

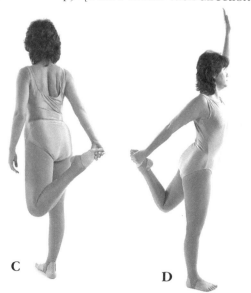

C　　　　D

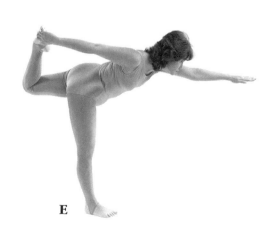

E

Tree Pose. *Improves posture, poise, balance, concentration, respiration; strengthens legs.* Stare at one spot on the wall or floor in front of you (but keep your head straight). Breathing normally, slowly raise your right leg and place it as high on the inside of your left leg as possible (**A**). Position your foot so your toes point down, and relax the leg; both these suggestions will help keep your foot from slipping down your leg. When you feel steady, exhale completely, then slowly breathe in and raise both arms over your head. Straighten your arms and place your palms together (**B**). Now relax your breath and hold the pose for a count of three. Watch for tightness in your stomach muscles which will tense your breathing. Relax your breath throughout. Keep staring at one spot for balance. If you have trouble balancing, practice this exercise standing next to a sturdy chair or the wall, and hold on with one hand. It's more important to relax your breath in this balance pose than to raise your arms overhead. If you are very limber and your back is strong, you may try the exercise with your ankle resting on the thigh (**C**). [3 times each side]

Cat Breath. *Limbers lower and midback; tightens stomach muscles; improves breathing.* Start on hands and knees. Breathe in, arch your back, and look up (**D**), so you feel the stretch all along your spine from tailbone to neck. Hold for a count of three. Then breathe out, round your back, and pull up on your stomach to increase the forward stretch (**E**). Tuck your chin and hold for a count of three. [3 repetitions]

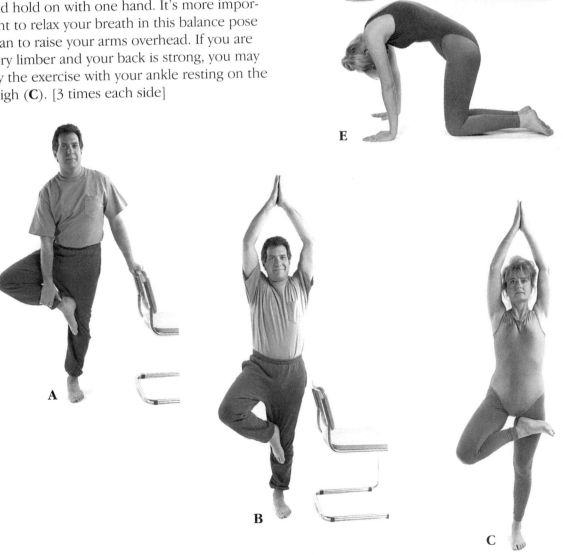

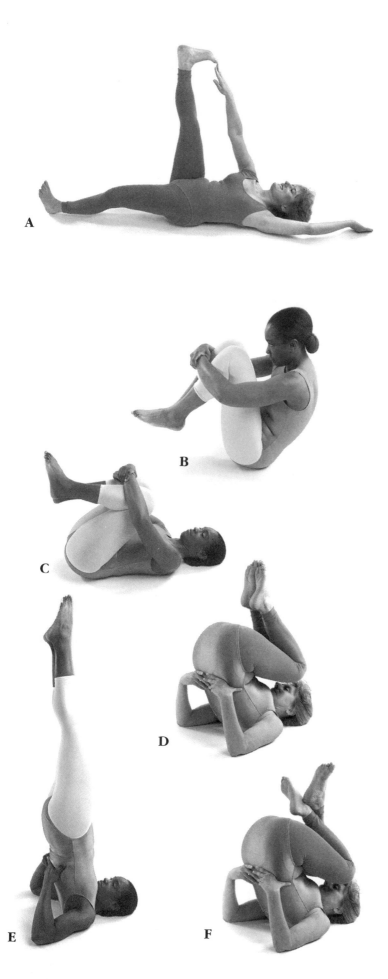

Alternate Toe Touch. *Stimulates nerves and muscles in the hips and pelvis; strengthens the legs and lower back.* Lie on your back with legs together and arms overhead on the floor. Breathe out completely, then breathe in and raise your left arm and left leg (**A**). Try to touch your toes, keeping your legs straight and without lifting your shoulder off the floor. Hold for a count of three. Breathe out and lower the leg and arm. Repeat with the right leg and arm. [3 times each side, alternating]

Shoulder Stand. *Stimulates thyroid and parathyroid; enhances function of all vital organs; relieves tension on heart and lungs; relaxes nervous system; removes fatigue.* If you have a disk problem in your neck, do not do this exercise; substitute the Easy Bridge (p. 116) instead. Start by sitting with knees drawn up to chest and arms wrapped around knees (**B**). Gently roll back and forth a few times (**C**) to make sure that the spine is in place with no pinched nerves or strained muscles. Then roll back, keeping knees to forehead, and immediately support your lower back with your hands and keep your knees bent and your body in the rounded position (**D**). Hold this position until you feel steady, then slowly straighten your legs toward the ceiling (**E**). If your legs appear to be more at a 45° angle, move your hands down your back toward the floor, push gently, and tuck your chin into your chest; your legs should straighten a bit more. Fix your gaze on the ceiling in the space between your big toes. Relax your breath. Hold for a count of three. As you get stronger, you can increase the hold to one-half minute, up to a full minute (do not exceed one minute). Women should not do this exercise during the menstrual period.

Come out of the pose by bending your knees and bringing them to your forehead. Cross your ankles (**F**) and slowly roll forward, rounding your back, until you come all the way up to a seated position. Bend forward for a few seconds to be sure the blood doesn't drain from your head too fast. [1 repetition]

Easy Cobra. *Gently limbers entire spine, balances both halves of body, improves circulation, massages all internal organs.* Lie on your stomach resting on your forearms with hands clasped and elbows on the floor just below your shoulders, fairly close to your body (**A**). Breathe out and let your head and upper back relax forward. Now breathe in and lift your head and eyes up and back as far as possible without strain, then continue breathing in, arching your back and stretching up on your elbows, so you feel a slight stretch along your entire spinal column (**B**). Do not strain. Hold for a count of three and do not blink. Breathe out and relax your back, then your head and eyes, until your forehead comes back down to your clasped hands. Caution: this exercise should not be done if you have had recent surgery or by women during the menstrual period, as it increases blood flow. [3 repetitions]

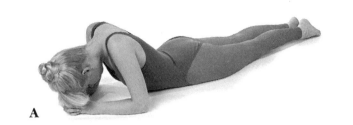

A

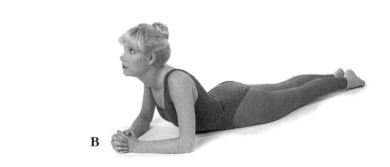

B

Boat Pose. *Strengthens back muscles, improves digestion and functioning of all internal organs.* Lie on your stomach, forehead to the floor and arms stretched out in front. Breathe out, then breathe in and lift your arms, legs, and head (**C**). Look up. Hold your breath and the position for a count of three, then breathe out and lower to your starting position. [3 repetitions]

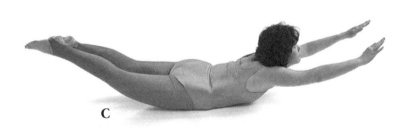

C

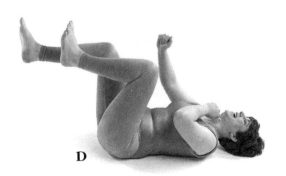

D

Laughasan. *Relieves muscle tension in the entire body; activates the immune system and releases endorphins.* Lie on your back and start pumping your legs as if you were riding a bicycle. Move your arms, too, and start to laugh. Pump your arms and legs as vigorously as you can and laugh out loud for at least 30 seconds (**D**). (This exercise can also be done in a chair.) Do this several times a day for a wonderful ebullient feeling.

Pain Management
Chapter 14

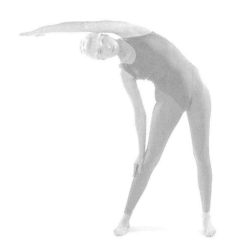

As many as a third of all Americans at some time in their lives suffer from some type of chronic pain. One source estimates that over 700 million work days are lost each year to chronic pain.

The unremitting stress of chronic pain affects all aspects of life. It often creates a cycle that begins with less and less physical activity, which results in more discouragement, leading to depression and even less activity. You feel trapped by your pain. Unrested, you feel irritable, you don't feel up to dealing with other people, you have difficulty becoming interested in or concentrating on anything except the pain, and you may develop a greater dependence on narcotics, alcohol, or other drugs. You may have developed automatic responses to pain that increase your withdrawal, depression, and fatigue.

Your brain naturally produces hormone-like chemicals, called endorphins, that closely resemble morphine. Endorphins seem to be a natural pain-control system, and are released as part of the brain's reaction to stress — but the supply is limited. Chronic stress, as experienced by those with chronic pain, may simply overwhelm the brain's ability to manufacture sufficient endorphins, leaving the individual even more vulnerable to the ravages of stress.

• *H*ow Yoga Can Help •

Many people do not realize that Yoga exercises and concentrative techniques were originally designed and practiced primarily to make the body healthy and strong so that one could live in a small space happily and sit immobile for meditation without discomfort. This fact has led to some ascetics using Yoga techniques to build endurance to pain (walking on hot coals, the "bed of nails," etc.). Although in most cases these "fakirs" have developed their skills for purposes of sideshow entertainment, it is true that Yoga techniques can help minimize the brain's acknowledgment of painful stimuli.

Yoga is one of the ways the body's supply of endorphins can be increased to help reduce pain naturally. Yoga also teaches stress-coping skills to help the body and brain conserve energy and recover faster. Using Yoga techniques for pain management can help minimize medication usage and help you lead a happier and fuller life. Yoga exercise, breathing, relaxation, and meditation techniques stimulate the body to produce more endorphins, distract the mind from pain, and reduce the tension that builds in muscles in reaction to pain. They teach effective stress-coping skills and provide an opportunity to "move through" the pain instead of resisting it, thereby reducing its full impact and allowing you to rest.

A simple routine of Yoga exercises stretches and relaxes large muscle groups, improves circulation and respiration, and stimulates the hormonal system. If you have been inactive for a long time because of pain, you'll need to start gradually with a minimum of three exercises a day until you are strong enough to do a full routine. (Note: If your chronic pain is due to arthritis or back or neck problems, see Chapters 4 and 6 for specific suggestions for those conditions.) It's important to exercise a little every day, as inactivity will only intensify the pain over time.

The Complete Breath, done seated or lying down in a comfortable position, focus your mind's attention on one point, namely, the sound of the breath as it is drawn in and out slowly, smoothly, and rhythmically. The intense focus of this exercise is a powerful tool for pain management. Because it is difficult to pay attention to the pain at the same time as you are concentrating on the sound of the breath, pain eventually recedes to the background or disappears altogether. As you learn, through Yoga, how to recognize harmful stress reactions, you learn to substitute healthier coping skills which include breathing techniques.

Relaxation training, a step-by-step process of relaxing each of your body's muscles in turn, helps to counteract your body's natural tendency to increase muscle tension in an unconscious effort to "push" the pain away — which only causes the pain to increase. Meditation training is a conscious effort to reduce your mind's constant chatter and to concentrate instead simply on the feeling of silence. Regular daily practice of meditation builds a foundation of internal strength by opening a door to a part of yourself that is not governed by the demands of your physical body, giving you a rest from the constant attention demanded by pain.

Yoga is highly effective in dealing with so-called "phantom pain" which occurs with the loss of a limb. In fantasy, one can learn to take the breath into the missing limb and ease the pain. Use the "I Love You" meditation technique (described on pp. 28-29) every day.

Most physicians recommend a multidisciplinary approach to chronic pain that uses several methods for relief including relaxation, gentle exercise, breathing, attention to diet, and guided imagery techniques. Yoga techniques can make the difference between a life ruled by pain and one in which pain plays only a "bit part."

• Special Concerns •

Resorting to drugs and alcohol for relief from chronic pain can lead to addiction, depression, and possibly confusion. These are dangerous methods and probably should be used only when absolutely necessary. Work closely with your physician to be sure that you are using the correct type and dosage of medication for your pain.

Persistent or severe pain can sometimes be a symptom of an underlying medical problem. Consult your physician to determine the cause of your pain, and ask him or her to help you choose which exercises are safe for you.

• Things You Can Do Throughout the Day •

Do the Complete Breath (see Chapter 1) whenever you feel yourself becoming anxious or obsessive about your pain or if you feel your muscles clenching in response to pain.

Take a 15-minute break and do a few exercises and a short relaxation and meditation session. It may be helpful to use a cassette tape (see Resources).

Gently massage your body to relax the muscles (see pp. 54-55).

Practice the "I Love You" meditation technique (pp. 28-29) to build acceptance of and love for your body.

• Dietary Suggestions •

By eating more nutritious foods, you can provide your body with the essential nutrients needed to activate its inner pain control system and to maximize its self-healing potential. Help reduce stress reactions and build up your supply of endorphins by feeding yourself a balanced, healthy diet. Make sure each meal has low-fat protein, fresh fruits and vegetables, and complex carbohydrates. Avoid sugary, high-fat, or artificially colored or flavored foods, overly processed foods, and caffeine and alcohol as much as possible. Allergic reactions to food additives, hypoglycemia from skipped meals, and the highs and lows of caffeine, alcohol, and excess sugar will increase your stress rather than reducing it. Many of our students find that daily multi-vitamin and mineral supplements help to provide the extra nutrients that you need when under stress. Extra calcium is a must for fighting pain, and vitamin C and the B complex are also very important. Check your diet carefully with an expert or consult a reputable book (see Appendix B, Further Reading).

• Daily Routine for Pain Management •

Start with the basic routine described in Chapter 1, then incorporate the special exercises in this chapter. These exercises have been chosen because they teach you how to stretch and relax your muscles, improve your concentration and blood circulation, compress the internal organs to stimulate hormone production, teach you to breathe better, and shift your focus from pain to the sound of the breath.

If you don't have time to do a full routine, or if your pain is so severe that you can't do a full routine at first, start with at least three warmup exercises and three of the exercises described below, and always do the full relaxation procedure and at least a few minutes of meditation. Best results will be obtained if you practice a little every day without fail.

Here is a list of the full sequence of techniques (including the basic routine):

Complete Breath, p. 26
Warmups, pp. 16-20
Side Stretch, p. 129
Dancer Pose, pp. 129-130
T Pose, p. 130
Standing Sun Pose, p. 21
Baby Pose, p. 24
Arm and Leg Balance, p. 130
Camel Pose, p. 131
Seated Sun Pose, p. 22
Tortoise Stretch, p. 23
Pigeon Pose, p. 131
Shoulder Stand, p. 132
Cobra Pose, p. 133
Relaxation and Meditation, pp. 26-27

Side Stretch. *Limbers back, legs, hips; limbers intercostal muscles (rib cage); improves respiration and balance; strengthens heart.* Stand with feet a comfortable distance apart, feet facing forward. Breathe in and raise your arms parallel to the floor (**A**), then breathe out and bend sideways to the left, sliding your left hand down your left thigh toward your knee. Grasp the leg firmly so you don't slip. Keeping your right arm as straight as possible, lift it over your head and as far toward the left as you can without strain (**B**). Eventually, your right arm should be parallel to the floor. Keep your body in a plane. Look straight ahead. Feel the stretch in the right ribs and hip. Hold for a count of three, then breathe in and come back up to the first position with arms outstretched. Make all movements smooth and easy; it's easy to overdo and strain by reaching too far down the leg. Keep both knees straight. [3 each side]

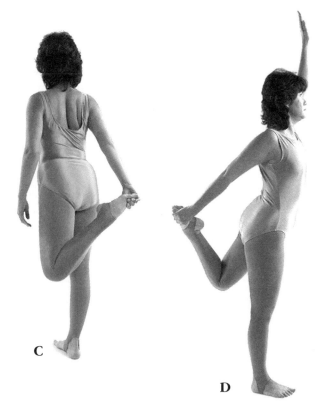

C

D

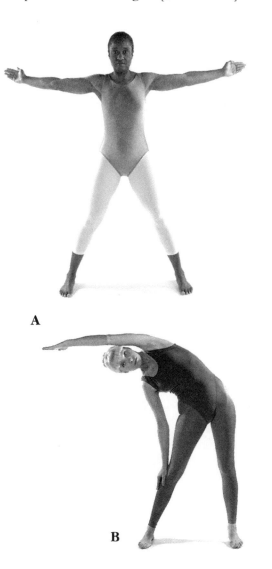

A

B

Dancer Pose. *Strengthens the lower back; limbers and strengthens the hips and thighs; improves mental poise; improves posture, balance, and concentration; strengthens ankles; relieves upper back tension.* Throughout the exercise, steady yourself by fixing your gaze on one spot on the wall in front of you. From a standing rest position, bend your right knee and grasp your right foot in back with your left hand (**C**). Check to be sure your stomach muscles are relaxed and your breathing steady. Slowly move into the completed Dancer Pose by raising your right arm straight up toward the ceiling so it is next to your ear and pulling your right leg up and back as far as possible without strain (**D**). Don't lean forward, and keep your supporting leg straight. Relax your stomach, breathe normally, and keep your gaze fixed on one spot. Hold for a count of three, then carefully return to the beginning position. [3 times each side]

Dancer Pose Extension. Try this extension after you have become proficient in the Dancer Pose. From the Dancer position after your 3-count hold as described above, maintain your gaze and, still breathing normally, slowly lower your body into the extended position (**A**). In addition to the benefits of the Dancer Pose, this variation stretches the back of the legs and increases strength and stamina. Keep your right leg as far up and back as possible. Your right arm extends straight ahead. Your left (supporting) leg remains straight. Stare at one spot for balance and hold for a count of three. Don't strain. Come back to a standing rest position.

T Pose. *Strengthens legs and back; improves vigor; tones abdominal organs; increases concentration, memory, and mental poise.* Start by holding on to a sturdy chair or counter for support. Stand about three feet away from the support and lean forward, keeping your neck straight so you are looking at the floor. Breathe in, balance on your left leg, and raise your right leg in back parallel to the floor — or as high as you can (**B**). Staring at one spot on the floor, let go of the support if you can and place your palms together (**C**). When you are in position, hold for a count of three, then breathe out and relax. [3 times each side]

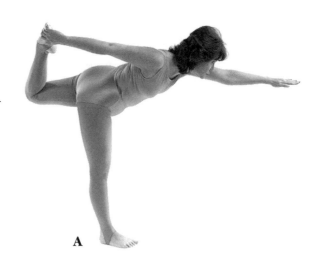

A

Arm & Leg Balance. *Strengthens muscles of the lower and midback, strengthens legs and hips; improves concentration.* On hands and knees, breathe out completely. Then breathe in and raise your left arm and right leg parallel to the floor (**D**). Look straight ahead at your outstretched arm, or, if your balance is shaky, stare at one spot on the floor. Hold for a count of three. Breathe out and lower. Repeat with the right arm and left leg. [3 each side, alternating opposites] If you feel very steady, you can vary this exercise by lifting the arm and leg on the same side of the body instead (**E**). [3 repetitions, each side]

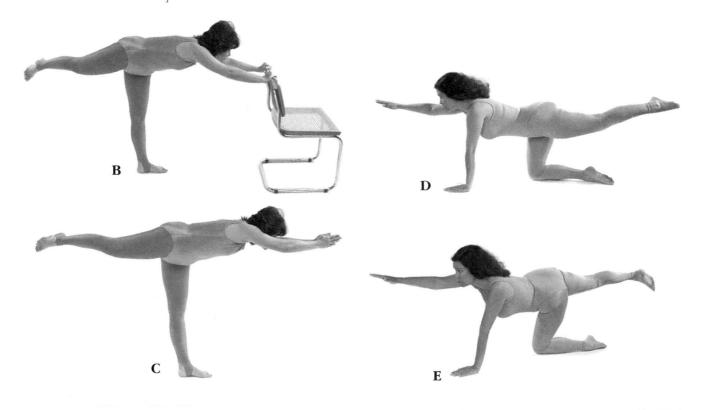

B

C

D

E

Camel Pose. *Limbers entire spine; improves circulation and respiration; stretches and strengthens thighs and knees; improves functioning of thyroid.* Kneel with legs slightly separated. The first two movements in this exercise help to prepare the spine for an intense stretch: Carefully bend back and grasp your left heel with your left hand. Push your hips forward slightly (**A**). Repeat on the right side. Now bend backward and grasp one heel with each hand. Push your hips forward as far as possible and let your head relax back (**B**) (unless you have neck problems, in which case do not let your head drop backward). Hold for a count of three. Release and rest briefly in the Baby Pose. As you get stronger, you can repeat if you wish. [1 repetition]

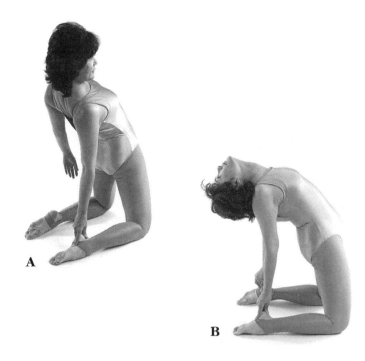

Pigeon Pose & Hold. *Stretches, strengthens, and tones spinal column, hip joints, and groin muscles; stimulates metabolic system; improves breathing.* From a kneeling position, slide your left leg straight back and sit on your right heel. Bend forward and rest your chest on your right thigh, and place your hands palms down on either side of your knee. Place your forehead on the floor and relax completely (**C**). Breathe out. Breathe in as you slowly curl your eyes, head, and chest up and back as far as you can comfortably (**D**). Hold for a count of three. Slowly breathe out as you curl down, bringing your chest down first, then your head and eyes. [3 repetitions]

After your third repetition, make fists and push your upper body up. Keep your legs and hips relaxed and your neck straight. Look at one spot on the floor. Tuck your left toes under. Hold for several seconds, breathing normally (**E**). Then switch sides: Push yourself up on all fours, stretching your right leg back straight and bringing your left leg forward. Repeat the entire sequence.

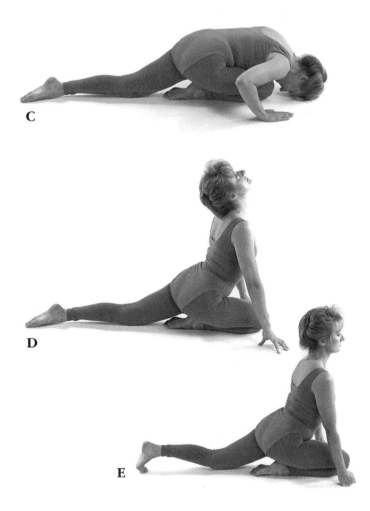

Shoulder Stand.   *Stimulates thyroid and parathyroid; enhances function of all vital organs; relieves tension on heart and lungs; relaxes nervous system; removes fatigue.* If you have a disk problem in your neck, do not do this exercise; substitute the Easy Bridge (p. 116) instead. Start by sitting with knees drawn up to chest and arms wrapped around knees (**A**). Gently roll back and forth a few times (**B**) to make sure that the spine is in place with no pinched nerves or strained muscles. Then roll back, keeping knees to forehead, and immediately support your lower back with your hands and keep your knees bent and your body in the rounded position (**C**). Hold this position until you feel steady, then slowly straighten your legs toward the ceiling (**D**). If your legs appear to be more at a 45° angle,

move your hands down your back toward the floor, push gently, and tuck your chin into your chest; your legs should straighten a bit more. Fix your gaze on the ceiling in the space between your big toes. Relax your breath. Hold for a count of three. As you get stronger, you can increase the hold to one-half minute, up to a full minute (do not exceed one minute). Women should not do this exercise during the menstrual period.

Come out of the pose by bending your knees and bringing them to your forehead. Cross your ankles (**E**) and slowly roll forward, rounding your back, until you come all the way up to a seated position. Bend forward for a few seconds to be sure the blood doesn't drain from your head too fast. [1 repetition]

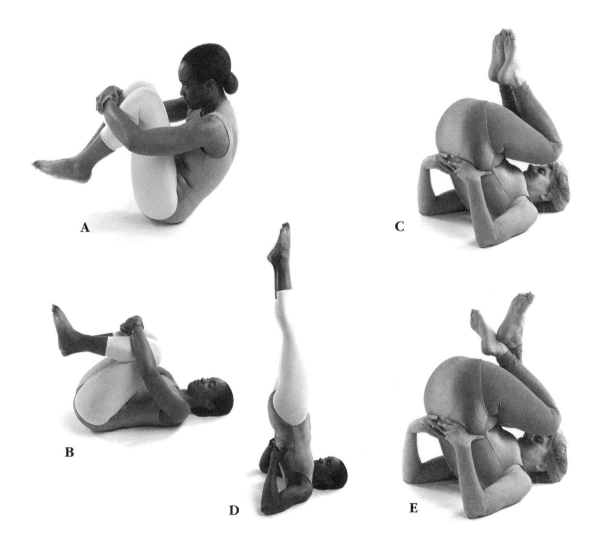

A

C

B

D

E

Cobra Pose. *Improves functioning of digestive, respiratory, and reproductive systems; limbers and strengthens entire spine; strengthens eyesight; equalizes two sides of body; improves complexion.* Lie on your stomach with legs together (those with occasional lower back trouble should separate the legs at first). Place your forehead on the floor and your palms down next to your armpits close to your body so your elbows point back and up, not out to the sides (**A**). Breathe out completely, then start to breathe in as you curl first your head and eyes back as far as they will go, then your chest, and then your stomach (**B**). Keep your hipbones on the floor — this is not a push-up — and your arms slightly bent (unless you are extremely limber). Use your back muscles more than your arms. Hold for a count of three at the top with your breath in and eyes looking up through your forehead. Do not blink. Then start to breathe out and curl forward slowly, in reverse: your stomach curls down first, then your chest, and finally your head and eyes. Your eyes are the first part of your body to curl up and the last to curl down. [3 repetitions]

Caution: This is a very powerful exercise and should not be done if you have had recent surgery or by women during the menstrual period, as it encourages blood flow.

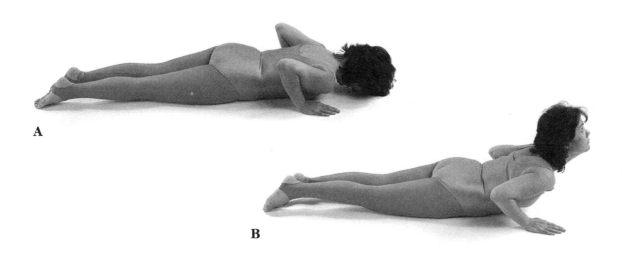

A

B

The Mental Effects of Yoga Exercise

Much of the benefit of Yoga exercises happens in your mind. It's as if your body takes a particular shape of an exercise and that position is imprinted on your brain where the healing properties of that exercise actually take effect. This is why it is so important to do each exercise exactly as instructed, to breathe correctly, to hold for the prescribed count, and to keep your attention on what you are doing at all times. This is also why you can achieve almost the same effects simply by imagining yourself doing the exercises. If you experience days on which you feel too ill to do any physical exercise, lie down, close your eyes, and imagine yourself going through your basic routine. Do at least three exercises in your mind, using the correct breathing pattern and repeating the exercise the prescribed number of times. Cultivating this ability to let your mind do most of the work will help in the management of pain by diverting your attention from pain. In addition, doing a meditation session and the "I Love You" technique at least once a day (preferably two times) will reinforce your mind's ability to relax you from the inside out.

*I*t is said that women are the more adaptable of the species. Whether that is true for every woman or not, it is true that women are more exposed to change simply because of the natural monthly physical and mental changes brought on by menstruation. From the time of puberty until menopause, women cope with changes in how they feel and look every month. For some women, these monthly changes in their bodies and emotions are slight and nearly unnoticeable; for others, the monthly course of menstruation is a dreaded ordeal — primarily because of the uncomfortable symptoms known as Premenstrual Syndrome (PMS).

The most common PMS symptoms are headaches, weight gain, bloating, fatigue, constipation, food cravings, and skin eruptions; irritability, tearfulness, tension, moodiness, and depression. Although medical science still doesn't know exactly what causes PMS in some women and not in others, it is believed that most of these symptoms result from fluctuations in hormone levels.

Menopause occurs naturally in every woman near the age of 50, when menstruation slows and then stops. For many women, this is seen as a time of new freedom, with more energy and focus for the fulfillment of life's ambitions. Others suffer at the prospect of loss of youth, children grown and gone, or dreams unfulfilled. Some women have trouble enjoying the positive aspects of menopause because of the hormonal changes, which can sometimes cause uncomfortable physical symptoms such as hot flashes, night sweats, vaginal dryness, mood swings, and anxiety. So-called "silent" changes in the body also occur during menopause, as the body reduces its production of estrogen; this increases a woman's risk of heart disease and osteoporosis.

It is sad that the process of aging has such negative connotations in our country, especially for women. Menopausal symptoms may be intensified because of the widespread belief that it is a period of decline and loss of status for women. In other parts of the world, menopause is heralded as the beginning of new opportunities for a productive, creative life free from the constraints of child-rearing. Women may take up roles involving more community leadership, or develop skills in the arts. Perhaps because menopause is seen in a more positive light, the physical symptoms may be noticed less.

Even if your symptoms are not severe, you should consult your physician regularly during menopause and take steps to protect yourself from the increased risks of heart disease and osteoporosis by exercising regularly. Make sure your diet is balanced, stop smoking if you haven't already, and practice stress management skills. Some women and their physicians turn to hormone replacement therapy automatically at menopause, while others try a more natural approach. Only you and your doctor will be able to make that decision.

A regular exercise program helps to counteract many of the effects of aging such as loss of muscle and bone mass, decline in heart and lung function, and joint stiffness. Exercise also improves posture, strengthens the immune system, raises endorphin levels, and increases blood flow to the body and brain.

• How Yoga Can Help •

The constellation of symptoms that result from shifting hormone levels every month during a woman's childbearing years, and during the process of menopause, can be greatly relieved by a daily program of Yoga exercise, breathing, and meditation.

Premenstrual Syndrome

A daily program of Yoga throughout the month will build a support system from the inside that will reduce the severity of PMS symptoms. Yoga exercises reduce muscle tension and help you become more centered and aware of your body. They improve posture and circulation so that all parts of your body and brain receive oxygen and other nutrients. Yoga has a direct effect on the body's chemistry by pressing on various glands and organs for a more balanced metabolism and the release of endorphins.

Breathing techniques will help you to concentrate better and to free yourself from anxious or fearful thoughts. You will find that you can use Yoga breathing exercises to reduce your stress reactions and maintain a steadier outlook on life.

Relaxation and meditation techniques are very important during this time to build emotional stability and to acknowledge your inner support system. When you experience the feeling of being happy within yourself, you will be less troubled by irritability, depression, and moodiness.

Menopause

One of the most important products of Yoga practice is an increase in self-esteem. In our culture, where youth and certain body shapes are held up as the ideal, women entering menopause often suffer greatly from loss of self-esteem. Yoga provides a positive reinforcement of the aging process by building self-awareness and raising self-esteem. The "I Love You" meditation technique (see Chapter 1) is ideal for this; through a systematic "flooding" of your body image with love and breath, you experience a new appreciation for who you are. Yoga helps reinforce the positive aspects of menopause by increasing your energy and stamina, improving posture and carriage so you feel better about how you look, and building an inner support system that will help you view the many changes in your life with anticipation instead of dread. Regular practice of meditation allows the cultivation of a more subtle part of yourself, which can bring to your later years a deep satisfaction and a continuing experience of growth.

A daily Yoga routine can help to alleviate many of the physical and emotional symptoms of menopause. Breathing and meditation techniques done just before retiring, and again if you wake during the night, can help you achieve a more restful sleep. Because Yoga exercises affect the body's chemistry, they can help reduce feelings of irritability, depression, and moodiness. Likewise, some Yoga exercises specifically stimulate the glandular and reproductive systems. Circulation is greatly improved with Yoga, so that all parts of the body receive oxygen and nutrients, and waste products are flushed out. Also, many Yoga exercises are weight-bearing (such as the Pigeon Pose, Plank, Shoulder Stand, and Easy Bridge) and therefore are beneficial in preventing and relieving osteoporosis. A regular Yoga program can also help you lose weight if you need to (see Chapter 16).

• Special Concerns •

See your physician regularly to monitor your symptoms and to rule out other conditions that may be causing them.

• Things You Can Do Throughout the Day •

If you are particularly troubled by mood swings, try to become more aware of your feelings throughout the day so that you can use a breathing or relaxation exercise when you want to stabilize your emotions or need to concentrate on some task.

Practice the "I Love You" meditation technique (see Chapter 1) daily to build self-confidence and self-esteem.

Learn coping skills to reduce harmful stress reactions. The Complete Breath is especially helpful anytime to relieve muscle tension in the stomach, face, shoulders, and back that will make your stress response worse.

• Dietary Suggestions •

Adult women of all ages need plenty of calcium. Most medical professionals, however, agree that the average American diet does not supply enough calcium, and that supplementation may be necessary. Dairy products, green leafy vegetables, tofu, and fortified orange juice are natural sources of calcium. It is now recognized that magnesium is needed in equal parts to calcium for optimum health. Foods rich in magnesium include wheat germ, almonds, cashews, and millet. High-quality calcium/magnesium supplements are also available.

Eliminating caffeine and alcohol can relieve many symptoms, especially headaches. Certain substances, such as hot drinks, caffeine, alcohol, and highly seasoned food, may act as triggers for hot flashes or other symptoms. Keeping a detailed record of what you eat for a week and what symptoms you experience will help you discover correlations that exist for you.

Recently there have been reports that estrogenlike substances in certain foods such as tofu and other soy products can be of great benefit to women. Many women have also experienced relief from menopausal symptoms with particular herbal preparations. Ask your physician or a competent nutritionist for more information.

• Daily Routine for PMS •

Start with the basic routine described in Chapter 1, then incorporate the special exercises in this chapter. These exercises gently stretch major muscle groups to release tension and ease lower back stiffness, regulate breathing, and improve circulation. They will also build concentration and strength, and stabilize emotions.

If you don't have time to do a full routine, do at least three warmup exercises and three of the exercises described below, and always do at least a few minutes of meditation. Best results will be obtained by practicing every day. We recommend that you not practice strenuous Yoga exercises (including those which compress the abdomen such as the Knee Squeeze, extreme backward bends such as the Cobra, or inverted exercises such as the Shoulder Stand) during the days when menstrual flow is heaviest — it could result in hemorrhage or extreme nervous upset. Instead, do a few simple warm-up exercises or stretches and spend extra time on relaxation and meditation.

Here is a list of the full sequence of techniques (including the basic routine):

Complete Breath, p. 26
Alternate Nostril Breath, p. 137
Warmups, pp. 16-20
Windmill, p. 137
Standing Sun Pose, p. 21
Baby Pose, p. 24
Seated Sun Pose, p. 22
Tortoise Stretch, p. 23
Pigeon Pose, p. 138
Diamond Pose, p. 138
Lower Back Stretch, p. 139
Easy Bridge, p. 139
Relaxation and Meditation, pp. 26-27

Alternate Nostril Breath.   *Balances both sides of body; improves concentration; strengthens respiration.* Using your right hand, curl your first and second fingers in toward your palm and hold them with the fleshy part of your thumb. Extend the fourth and fifth fingers straight. Start by closing your right nostril with your thumb (**A**) and breathe in through your left nostril. Breathe completely and slowly, just as in the Complete Breath. Then close your left nostril with the fourth and fifth fingers (**B**), and breathe out through your right nostril. Breathe in through the right nostril, then close with your thumb and breathe out, then in, through your left nostril. Continue for about 5 breath cycles to start (later you can add more repetitions if you wish). Focus on the sound of the breath. Breathe evenly and smoothly.

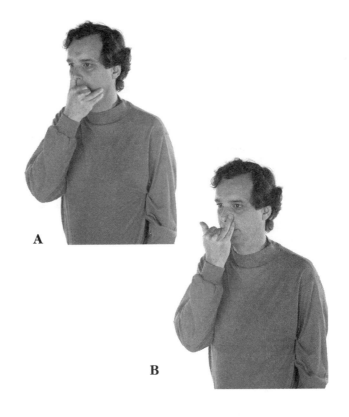

Windmill.   *Limbers and strengthens lower back, hip joints, and upper thigh; improves respiration; reduces waistline.* Stand with your feet as far apart as you can comfortably, toes pointed in. Place your hands on your lower back, thumbs over your hips and fingers supporting your lower back. Start by breathing in completely and turning toward the left (**C**). Breathe out as you bend your head toward your left leg (**D**) and continue moving over to your right leg. Now start to breathe in as you come back to a standing position and face front. Finish breathing in completely. Repeat twice more in the same direction. Your breathing pattern in this exercise follows the circular movement of your head: You are breathing out for two-thirds of the circle (from standing, over to the left leg, then to the right leg) and breathing in for the remaining third of the circle (as you stand up). [3 slow circles each direction]

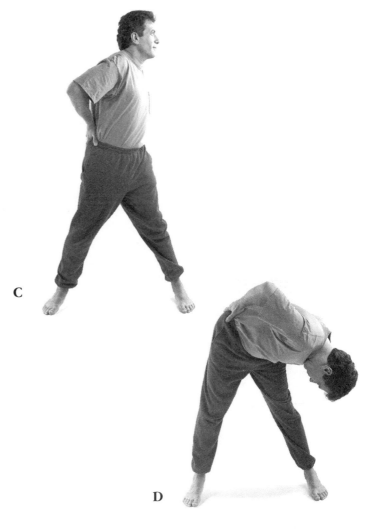

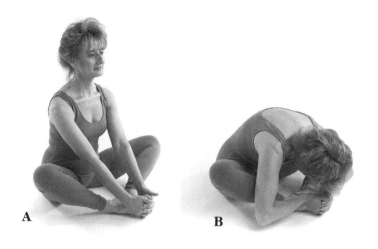

A   B

Diamond Pose. *Limbers lower back, hips and groin muscles; releases back tension; helps reduce abdomen.* Sit straight with knees bent and the soles of your feet touching. Grasp your ankles with both hands and rest your elbows on or above your thighs. Breathe in completely, then breathe out as you lean forward slightly and press down on your thighs with your arms. Hold for a count of three. Release and repeat twice more. Now lace your fingers around your toes, breathe in, and straighten your spine (**A**). Breathe out as you bend forward, letting your elbows fall outside your legs this time (**B**). Hold for a count of three, then breathe in and come back up. [3 repetitions]

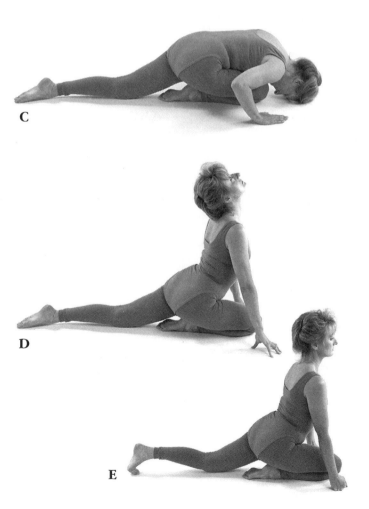

C
D
E

Pigeon Pose & Hold. *Stretches, strengthens, and tones spinal column, hip joints, and groin muscles; stimulates metabolic system; improves breathing.* From a kneeling position, slide your left leg straight back and sit on your right heel. Bend forward and rest your chest on your right thigh, and place your hands palms down on either side of your knee. Place your forehead on the floor and relax completely (**C**). Breathe out. Breathe in as you slowly curl your eyes, head, and chest up and back as far as you can comfortably (**D**). Hold for a count of three. Slowly breathe out as you curl down, bringing your chest down first, then your head and eyes. [3 repetitions]

After your third repetition, make fists and push your upper body up. Keep your legs and hips relaxed and your neck straight. Look at one spot on the floor. Tuck your left toes under (**E**). Hold for several seconds, breathing normally. Then switch sides: Push yourself up on all fours, stretching your right leg back straight and bringing your left leg forward. Repeat the entire sequence.

Lower Back Stretch.   *Improves functioning of internal organs. Improves circulation; strengthens and limbers the shoulders, back, and hip joints; helps to trim the waistline.* If you have a spinal disk problem, be very careful with this exercise. Lie on your back with your legs together and arms stretched out to the sides, palms down. Breathe out, then breathe in as you lift your left leg and hook your left toe under your right knee. Breathe out as you bend your left leg to the right over your right leg toward the floor as far as possible without straining (**A**). Keep your shoulders and arms on the floor and keep your right leg straight. Hold the position and your breath for a count of three. Breathe in as you roll back, lift your left knee up, and straighten your leg toward the ceiling. Breathe out as you return the leg to the floor. [3 times each side, alternating]

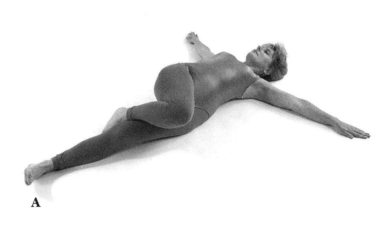

A

Easy Bridge.   *Improves functioning of thyroid; eases back pain and fatigue; increases circulation to head; helps relieve bedsores.* Lying on your back, bend your knees and bring your feet as close to your hips as possible. Separate your feet several inches. Place your arms palms down at your sides. Relax your neck and upper back, breathe out completely, pushing your waist to the floor slightly, then breathe in and raise your hips, curling up just to your waist (**B**) (your back will be rounded and your chin tucked toward your chest). Hold for a count of three, then breathe out and lower. Next, breathe in and lift your hips as high as you can without strain, keeping your shoulders on the floor and arching your back (**C**). Your chin will be tucked into your chest. Hold for a count of three, then slowly lower and breathe out. As you become more limber, you can hold onto your ankles for a greater stretch. [3 repetitions each variation]

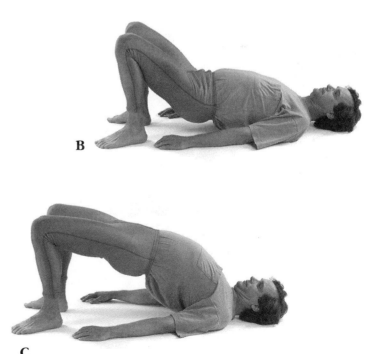

B

C

• *D*aily Routine for Menopause •

Start with the basic routine described in Chapter 1, then incorporate the special exercises in this chapter. These exercises stimulate the glandular and reproductive systems, resulting in a more balanced alignment of body chemistry and easing the symptoms caused by drastic hormone fluctuations. The gentle weight-bearing exercises in this routine will help to prevent loss of bone mass. These exercises also improve circulation, help to balance metabolism, prevent memory loss, and build steadiness of mind.

If you don't have time to do a full routine, do at least three warmup exercises and three of the exercises described below, and always do at least a few minutes of meditation. Best results will be obtained by practicing every day.

Here is a list of the full sequence of techniques (including the basic routine):

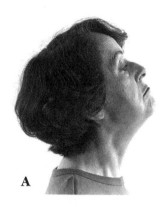

A

Throat Stretches.   *Keeps neck muscles strong and limber; prevents aging of the skin of the face and throat; helps to improve circulation to the brain.* With lips and teeth together, breathing normally, jut your chin forward, gently tensing the muscles under your chin (**A**), then retract your head to normal position, and relax your neck. Then turn your head toward the right and repeat: jut your chin forward, gently pushing without straining your neck. You'll feel a slight pull, but be careful not to go too far. Then retract, relax, and come back to the center position. Repeat the stretch, then turn toward the left and repeat. [3 times each direction, inserting a middle point stretch each time]

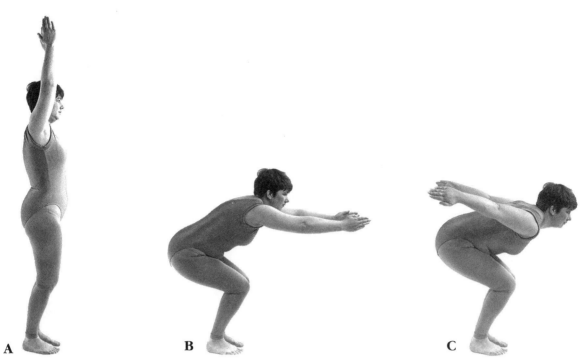

A   B   C

Swing Stretch.   *Improves circulation; limbers the back and legs.* Standing with feet slightly separated and arms at sides, breathe in and stretch your arms forward and up as far as you can (**A**), then breathe out, bend your knees, and swing your arms down in front (**B**) and all the way back (**C**). Breathe in and swing back up with arms overhead, straightening your knees. Move with the breath. Stretch up as far as possible each time. [3 or more repetitions]

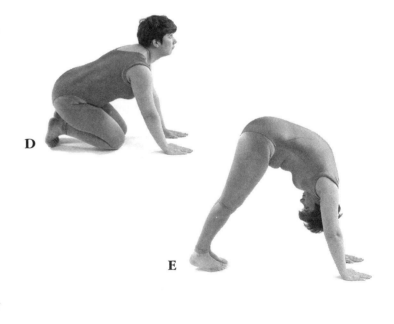

D

E

Stretching Dog.   *Limbers lower back and hips; stretches back of legs; increases circulation to head; strengthens heart.* Sit on your heels, toes tucked under and hands on the floor a few inches in front of your knees. Breathe in and arch your back, looking up (**D**). Hold for a count of three. Breathe out and straighten your legs, pushing your body into a V position (**E**). Tuck your chin toward your chest and hold for a count of three. [3 repetitions]

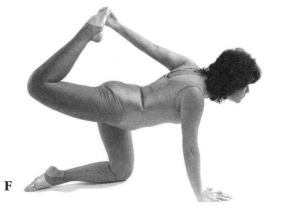

F

Bow Variation.   *Strengthens vertebrae, back and shoulder muscles, and hips and thighs; improves balance and memory.* Start on hands and knees, with hands on the floor directly beneath your shoulders. Reach back with your right hand and grasp your left foot. Breathe in as you lift the foot up away from your body, arching your back a little (**F**). Hold for a count of three. Breathe out and relax. [3 times each side, alternating]

Thigh Stretch.   *Stretches all muscles of the legs and hips; improves respiration; increases circulation.* Stand with feet apart a comfortable distance and swivel to face left. Bend forward and place your hands on either side of your left foot. Bend your left leg, lower your hips, breathe in, arch your back and look up (**A**). Hold for a count of three. Now breathe out and straighten your legs, keeping the toes of your left foot pointed and tucking your head in toward your left leg (**B**). Hold for a count of three. [3 each side]

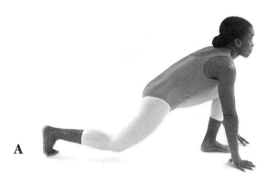

A

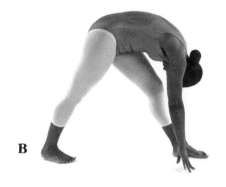

B

Plank Pose.   *Strengthens arms, shoulders, and neck; improves circulation in upper body; strengthens back.* From hands and knees, straighten your legs and position your hips so your legs and torso are in a straight line. Lean on your left hand and stretch your right hand out in front, gazing at your fingers (**C**). Hold for a quick count of three, then switch sides. If you are not strong enough to support your weight entirely on one hand, start by supporting yourself on alternate forearms instead, or simply lean on one hand, then the other, without raising the other arm off the floor, until you get stronger. [3 times each side]

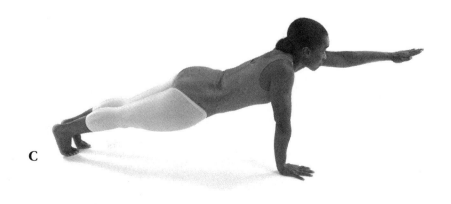

C

Shoulder Stand.   *Stimulates thyroid and parathyroid; enhances function of all vital organs; relieves tension on heart and lungs; relaxes nervous system; removes fatigue.* If you have a disk problem in your neck, do not do this exercise; substitute the Easy Bridge (p. 139) instead. Start by sitting with knees drawn up to chest and arms wrapped around knees (**A**). Gently roll back and forth a few times (**B**) to make sure that the spine is in place with no pinched nerves or strained muscles. Then roll back, keeping knees to forehead, and immediately support your lower back with your hands and keep your knees bent and your body in the rounded position (**C**). Hold this position until you feel steady, then slowly straighten your legs toward the ceiling (**D**). If your legs appear to be more at a 45° angle, move your hands down your back toward the floor, push gently, and tuck your chin into your chest; your legs should straighten a bit more. Fix your gaze on the ceiling in the space between your big toes. Relax your breath. Hold for a count of three. As you get stronger, you can increase the hold to one-half minute, up to a full minute (do not exceed one minute). Women should not do this exercise during the menstrual period.

Come out of the pose by bending your knees and bringing them to your forehead. Cross your ankles (**E**) and slowly roll forward, rounding your back, until you come all the way up to a seated position. Bend forward for a few seconds to be sure the blood doesn't drain from your head too fast. [1 repetition]

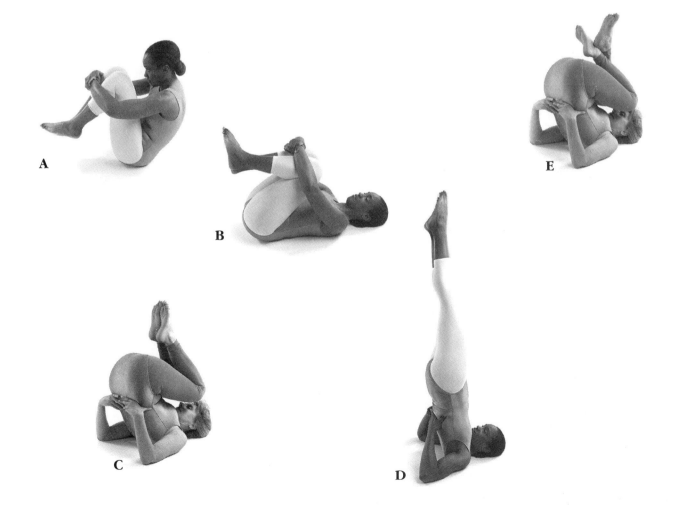

A

B

C

D

E

Cobra Pose.   *Improves functioning of digestive, respiratory, and reproductive systems; limbers and strengthens entire spine; strengthens eyesight; equalizes two sides of body; improves complexion.* Lie on your stomach with legs together (those with occasional lower back trouble should separate the legs at first). Place your forehead on the floor and your palms down next to your armpits close to your body so your elbows point back and up, not out to the sides (**A**). Breathe out completely, then start to breathe in as you curl first your head and eyes back as far as they will go, then your chest, and then your stomach (**B**). Keep your hipbones on the floor — this is not a push-up — and your arms slightly bent (unless you are extremely limber). Use your back muscles more than your arms. Hold for a count of three at the top with your breath in and eyes looking up through your forehead. Do not blink. Then start to breathe out and curl forward slowly, in reverse: your stomach curls down first, then your chest, and finally your head and eyes. Your eyes are the first part of your body to curl up and the last to curl down.
[3 repetitions]

Caution: This is a very powerful exercise and should not be done if you have had recent surgery or by women during the menstrual period, as it encourages blood flow.

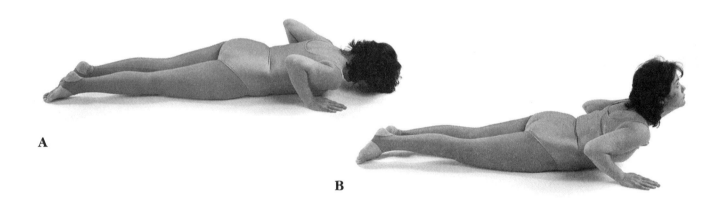

A

B

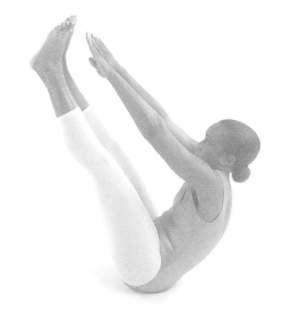

Most people feel better and look better when they are close to their optimum weight. Excess weight can result in feelings of depression, lack of self-esteem, anxiety, and feelings of inadequacy. But more importantly, maintaining optimum weight is healthier: Excess weight raises the risks for adult-onset diabetes, hypertension, and coronary artery disease, among other problems, and can even contribute to arthritis and back pain. These conditions are particularly likely to develop if you are also over 35 years of age.

As our bodies age, our metabolism naturally slows down. This is due to many causes, among them less efficient hormone production by the thyroid gland, loss of muscle tissue, and a slower recovery rate from the hormonal changes produced by the body's response to stress. Those with a sedentary lifestyle are particularly likely to gain weight as they grow older unless they exercise more and adjust their diet to include less fat.

Most weight-control experts have very simple advice: eat less and exercise more. It is possible — and even desirable — to adjust your diet so that you still eat the foods you enjoy; you simply learn to reduce portions. If you combine this with more regular exercise, you will lose fat and build muscle. Exercise not only uses up calories by itself, it also stimulates the body's metabolic rate so that calories are burned at a higher rate even at rest, enabling you to reach and maintain an ideal weight faster and better than dieting alone. Exercise has many more benefits, of course,

among them protection against heart disease, greater joint limberness, greater elasticity of the blood vessels, and stronger bones.

Losing weight does not need to be a painful punishment that you inflict on yourself. Diets and exercise programs that are based on self-hate and suffering will almost certainly fail when the feeling of deprivation becomes too much to bear. Yoga stresses non-violence to yourself; with this outlook, you will be able to follow a balanced program that helps you develop the skills to achieve your goals without causing yourself — or anyone else — to suffer.

• *H*ow Yoga Can Help •

Yoga is a gentle way to bring a balanced attitude to all aspects of life. It can help you control your weight more effectively by encouraging concentration and strengthening willpower. The techniques of Yoga are enjoyable ways to change your attitudes about exercise, diet, and self-image.

People who hate to exercise usually don't do it regularly. Yoga exercise is self-motivating because, after a short time of regular practice, the body actually enjoys Yoga exercises. The exercises in this chapter are more vigorous than the usual routine, and, although they will not take off inches as fast as more strenuous exercise, they will improve your shape by stabilizing metabolism, improving posture and circulation, and toning muscles in the back, stomach, and legs. As muscle tension is released and flexibility increased, you will feel more relaxed and poised. As your personality becomes quieter and freer from the demands of stress, you'll find more time to pay attention to inner feelings, needs, and thoughts. This makes for a more complete, balanced person who can face stress with greater ease and strength.

Many overweight people automatically reach for food as an escape from stress and for immediate comfort. Yoga helps change these reactions by replacing food with a breathing or exercise technique during periods of stress. You no longer want to harm yourself with destructive eating habits.

The relaxation and meditation aspects of Yoga support all your behavioral goals. Regular practice of meditation builds concentration and willpower, helping you stick to calorie or portion allotments or to a regular daily exercise program. Meditation also may help stimulate insight into the unconscious motivators of your eating behavior.

The "I Love You" meditation technique described in Chapter 1 is an invaluable aid for anyone on a weight control program. Do it every day to build your self-confidence and help you feel better about yourself as you change your lifestyle and image.

• Special Concerns •

Try to avoid an "all-or-nothing" approach to weight loss. The easiest way to "backslide" is to reason that if you can't do the program perfectly and completely, then it's not worth doing at all. This is a fallacy. If you regularly practice something every day — even if it's just a few exercises and a few minutes of meditation — you will maintain the continuity and momentum that will build success in Yoga practice.

• Things You Can Do Throughout the Day •

When you find yourself craving the wrong kind of food, substitute a few exercises. If you're at work or otherwise without privacy, do a few Complete Breaths to relax your mind and body and take your mind off the craving. Carry some nutritious food with you at all times so that if you can't help eating, you will eat the right type of food.

• Dietary Suggestions •

As mentioned above, you don't have to completely eliminate your favorite foods, even if they are high in fat. In fact, cutting out these foods entirely leads to cravings and often results in binges. This is why drastic short-term diets seldom keep the weight off. Such starvation diets actually lower metabolism even further as the body tries to compensate for not receiving enough fuel. It is much healthier — and will keep you happier — to lose weight more gradually by changing eating habits and exercising more.

For some of the same reasons, avoid diet pills and fasting. Yoga provides a type of self-motivation that doesn't come in a pill. When you change your outlook to one of self-care, the things you do for yourself — exercise, good nutrition, getting enough rest — don't seem like suffering; instead, they make you happy. Fasting is discouraged in Yoga because it is considered a form of violence to the body. In Yoga, develop the idea that your body is your friend, not your enemy; if you treat it with respect, it will support you in everything you need to do.

Consult a reputable nutritionist or your physician for a weight-reducing diet that is right for you. Most healthy diet plans include adequate protein, are low in fat, and are high in fruits, vegetables, and complex carbohydrates.

• *D*aily Routine for Weight Management •

Start with the basic routine described in Chapter 1, then incorporate the special exercises in this chapter. These exercises have been chosen because they improve concentration and willpower, enhance the ability to relax, improve heart and lung conditioning, teach stress-coping skills, and enhance self-esteem.

If you don't have time to do a full routine, do at least three warmup exercises and three of the exercises described below, and always do at least a few minutes of meditation. Best results will be obtained by practicing every day.

Here is a list of the full sequence of techniques (including the basic routine):

Complete Breath, p. 26
Warmups, pp. 16-20
Alternate Triangle, p. 148
Side Stretch, p. 148
T Pose, p. 149
Cobra V-Raise, p. 149
Standing Sun Pose, p. 21
Baby Pose, p. 24
Seated Sun Pose, p. 22
Tortoise Stretch, p. 23
Plank Pose, p. 149
Big Sit-Up, p. 150
Lower Back Stretch, p. 150
Walk, p. 150
Shoulder Stand, p. 151
Airplane Series, p. 152
Relaxation and Meditation, pp. 26-27

Alternate Triangle. *Stretches and strengthens muscles in the back, hips, and shoulders; compresses internal organs, stimulating metabolism; improves circulation to legs and feet.* With legs separated as far as is comfortable and toes pointed forward, breathe in and raise your arms straight out to the sides horizontally (**A**). Breathe out and stretch to the left reaching down your left leg with both hands. Grasp the leg firmly and pull gently by bending your elbows (**B**) (if you can't bend your elbows, grasp higher on the leg toward your knee; it's more important to pull with your arms [to avoid straining your back muscles] than it is to reach further down your leg). Tuck your head and hold your breath out for a count of three. Breathe in as you slowly straighten and bring your arms back into the outstretched position. [3 times each side]

Side Stretch. *Limbers back, legs, hips; limbers intercostal muscles (rib cage); improves respiration and balance; strengthens heart.* Stand with feet a comfortable distance apart, feet facing forward. Breathe in and raise your arms parallel to the floor (**A**), then breathe out and bend sideways to the left, sliding your left hand down your left thigh toward your knee. Grasp the leg firmly so you don't slip. Keeping your right arm as straight as possible, lift it over your head and as far toward the left as you can without strain (**C**). Eventually, your right arm should be parallel to the floor. Keep your body in a plane. Look straight ahead. Feel the stretch in the right ribs and hips. Hold for a count of three, then breathe in and come back up to the first position with arms outstretched. Make all movements smooth and easy; it's easy to overdo and strain by reaching too far down the leg. Keep both knees straight; it's more important to keep the legs straight than to reach the ankle. [3 each side]

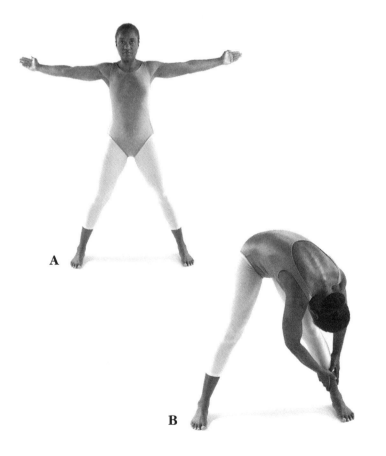

A

B

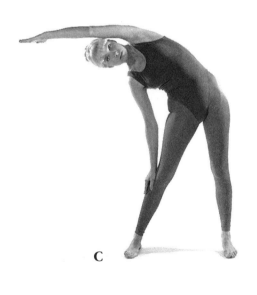

C

T Pose. *Strengthens legs and back; improves vigor; tones abdominal organs; increases concentration, memory, and mental poise.* Start by holding on to a sturdy chair or counter for support. Stand about three feet away from the support and lean forward, keeping your neck straight so you are looking at the floor. Breathe in, balance on your left leg, and raise your right leg in back parallel to the floor — or as high as you can (**A**). Staring at one spot on the floor, release the support and place palms together. When you are in position, hold for a count of three, then breathe out and relax. [3 times each side]

Cobra V-Raise. *Strengthens legs, back, shoulders, and rib cage; strengthens heart; improves functioning of the organs in the pelvic region; reduces body fat.* Walk your hands forward on the floor, keeping your heels down as far as possible, until your hands are about 4 to 5 feet in front of you. Tuck your chin into your chest and breathe out. This is the "V" position (**C**). Now, keeping your arms straight, breathe in and slowly lower your body, arching your back and looking up and back (**D**) (the "cobra" position). Hold for a count of three. Push back slowly into the V position, breathing out and tucking your chin into your chest. Hold for a count of three. [3 repetitions]

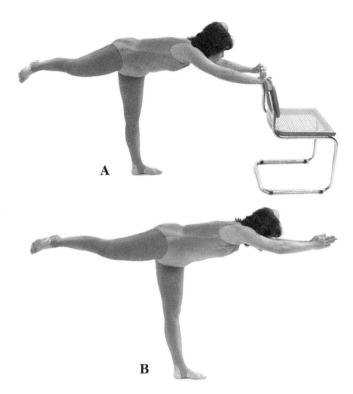

A

B

Plank Pose. *Strengthens arms, shoulders, and neck; improves circulation in upper body; strengthens back.* From hands and knees, straighten your legs and position your hips so your legs and torso are in a straight line. Lean on your left hand and stretch your right hand out in front, gazing at your fingers (**E**). Hold for a quick count of three, then switch sides. If you are not strong enough to support your weight entirely on one hand, start by supporting yourself on alternate forearms instead, or simply lean on one hand, then the other, without raising the other arm off the floor, until you get stronger. [3 times each side]

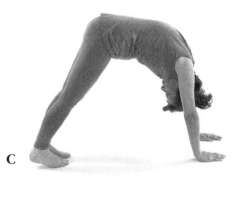

C

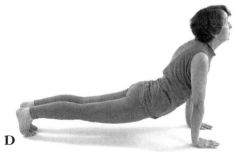

D

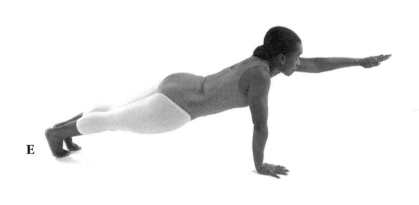

E

Big Sit-Up. *Strengthens abdominal and leg muscles; improves balance and concentration; relieves constipation and urinary tract difficulties.* Lie on your back with arms over your head and legs together. Breathe in and lift your arms, legs, and upper body at the same time (**A**). Balancing on the end of your spine, reach to touch your toes, keeping your legs straight. Hold for a quick count of three, then relax and breathe out. [3 repetitions]

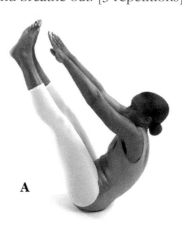

A

Lower Back Stretch. *Improves functioning of internal organs. Improves circulation; strengthens and limbers the shoulders, back, and hip joints; helps to trim the waistline.* If you have a spinal disk problem, be very careful with this exercise. Lie on your back with your legs together and arms stretched out to the sides, palms down. Breathe out, then breathe in as you lift your left leg and hook your left toe under your right knee. Breathe out as you bend your left leg to the right over your right leg toward the floor as far as possible without straining (**C**). Keep your shoulders and arms on the floor and keep your right leg straight. Hold the position and your breath for a count of three. Breathe in as you roll back, lift your left knee up, and straighten your leg toward the ceiling. Breathe out as you return the leg to the floor. [3 times each side, alternating]

Walk. *Reduces body fat from hips, thighs, and buttocks; strengthens legs, lower back, and abdomen.* Lie on your back with arms at your sides, palms down. Raise your legs straight up and flex your feet toward your face. "Walk" your legs back and forth (**B**), keeping the legs straight, for several seconds, breathing normally, then relax and lower your legs to the floor slowly.

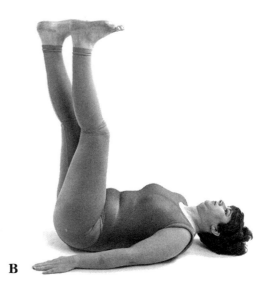

B

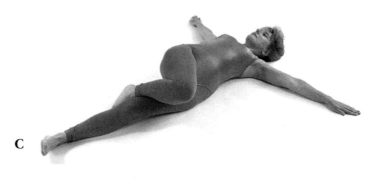

C

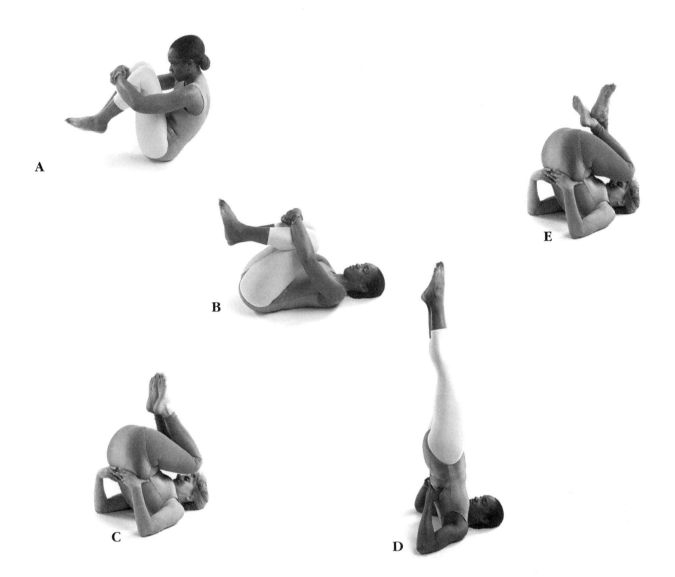

Shoulder Stand. *Stimulates thyroid and parathyroid; enhances function of all vital organs; relieves tension on heart and lungs; relaxes nervous system; removes fatigue.* If you have a disk problem in your neck, do not do this exercise; substitute the Easy Bridge (p. 116) instead. Start by sitting with knees drawn up to chest and arms wrapped around knees (**A**). Gently roll back and forth a few times (**B**) to make sure that the spine is in place with no pinched nerves or strained muscles. Then roll back, keeping knees to forehead, and immediately support your lower back with your hands and keep your knees bent and your body in the rounded position (**C**). Hold this position until you feel steady, then slowly straighten your legs toward the ceiling (**D**). If your legs appear to be more at a 45° angle,

move your hands down your back toward the floor, push gently, and tuck your chin into your chest; your legs should straighten a bit more. Fix your gaze on the ceiling in the space between your big toes. Relax your breath. Hold for a count of three. As you get stronger, you can increase the hold to one-half minute, up to a full minute (do not exceed one minute). Women should not do this exercise during the menstrual period.

Come out of the pose by bending your knees and bringing them to your forehead. Cross your ankles (**E**) and slowly roll forward, rounding your back, until you come all the way up to a seated position. Bend forward for a few seconds to be sure the blood doesn't drain from your head too fast. [1 repetition]

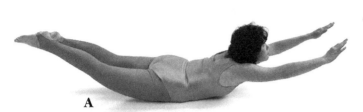

A

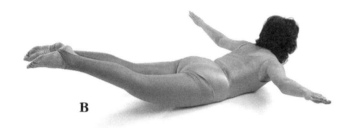

B

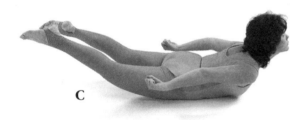

C

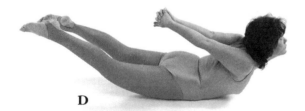

D

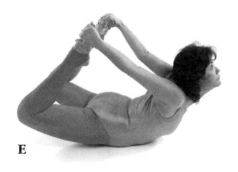

E

Airplane Series. *Strengthens entire spine; massages internal organs; improves breathing; strengthens shoulders, hips, and thighs.* This is a very challenging sequence but one which will give you a great deal of energy and strength. Lie on your stomach with arms overhead and forehead on the floor. Breathe in and lift your arms, legs, and head as in the Boat Pose (**A**). Hold for a quick count of three, then relax and breathe out, bringing your arms out sideways as in the Swan Dive. Breathe in and lift (**B**), holding for a count of three, then relax and breathe out, bringing your arms down to your sides. Breathe in and lift again (**C**), hold, then breathe out and relax, clasping your hands behind you. Breathe in and lift (**D**), hold, then relax and breathe out, grasping both ankles or feet. Breathe in and lift as in the Bow Pose (**E**), hold, then relax and breathe out. [1-3 repetitions]

Combining Yoga with Other Types of Exercise

As part of a weight-loss program (or any general fitness program) you may choose to practice some more vigorous types of exercise for aerobic conditioning. The best choices, according to the principles of Yoga, are those that work on both sides of the body equally, such as walking, running, swimming, and cycling — as opposed to sports like tennis, which use your dominant side almost exclusively. Your Yoga exercise routine can be a very effective warm-up and cool-down routine before and after exercising. We recommend that you do your meditation session after exercising, however, so that you give yourself time to internalize the quiet feelings that you experience in meditation.

The following exercises can be done in a chair. Use a straight, sturdy chair. Your feet should be firmly placed on the floor for support.

All breathing techniques, pp. 24-26, 96, 137
Arm Reach, p. 61
Arm Swing, p. 61
Arm Circles, p. 16
Baby Pose, p. 52
Elbow Roll, p. 53
Elbow Twist, p. 17
Eye Palming, p. 48
Foot Flap and Ankle Rotation, p. 54
Frog Pose, p. 105
Full Bend, p. 19 (Sit with knees apart, feet flat on the floor, and hips pressed against the chair back.)
Knee Squeeze, p. 107
Laughasan, p. 28
Lion Pose, p. 96
Massage, pp. 54-55
Neck Stretch, p. 17
Shoulder Roll, p. 16
Spine Twist, p. 107
Throat Stretches, p. 140
Relaxation and Meditation, pp. 26-27

The following exercises can be done in bed.

All breathing techniques, pp. 24-26, 96, 137
Alternate Toe Touch, p. 124
Boat Pose, p. 49
Cobra Pose, p. 39
Diamond Pose, p. 114
Easy Bridge, p. 64
Easy Cobra Pose, p. 57
Floor Stretch, p. 71
Foot Flap and Ankle Rotation, p. 54
Knee Squeeze, p. 38
Laughasan, p. 28
Lion Pose, p. 96
Lower Back Stretch, p. 48
Massage, pp. 54-55
Pelvic Twist, p. 98
Seated Sun Pose, p. 22
Swan Dive, p. 39
Throat Stretches, p. 140
Tortoise Stretch, p. 23
Walk, p. 150
Relaxation and Meditation, pp. 26-27

Further Reading
Appendix B

Books, articles, and other resources pertaining to each of the health topics covered in this book are listed below by chapter. An asterisk (*) indicates that the book is not currently in print but may still be available in your local library.

Chapter 1: Getting a Head Start on Health

Consumer Reports on Health. Monthly newsletter published by Consumers Union, 101 Truman Ave., Yonkers, NY 10703-1057.

Davis, Adelle. *Let's Get Well.* Harcourt, Brace & World, 1965.

Davis, Adelle. *Let's Stay Healthy: A Guide to Lifelong Nutrition.* New American Library/Dutton, 1983.

Null, Gary. *The Complete Guide to Health and Nutrition.* Dell, 1986.

Nutrition Action. Monthly newsletter published by the Center for Science in the Public Interest, Suite 300, 1875 Connecticut Avenue NW, Washington, DC.

Walnut Acres (mail-order firm for natural foods). Penns Creek, PA 17862; (800) 433-3998.

Chapter 2: Addiction

Kasl, Charlotte Davis. *Many Roads, One Journey, Moving Beyond the 12 Steps.* Harper Collins (No date).

Peele, Stanton, with Archie Brodsky. *The Truth About Addiction and Recovery.* Simon & Schuster, 1992.

Porterfield, Kay Marie. *Focus On Addictions: A Reference Handbook.* ABC-CL10, 1992.

Steffens, Bradley. *Addiction.* Greenhaven Press, 1994.

Chapter 3: Anxiety

Anxiety Disorders Association of America, 6000 Executive Blvd., Rockville, MD 20852; (301) 231-9350.

Council on Anxiety Disorders, P.O. Box 17011, Winston-Salem, NC 27116; (919) 722-7760.

Marks, Isaac M. *Living With Fear.* McGraw-Hill, 1978.

Matsakis, Aphrodite. *I Can't Get Over It.* New Harbinger Publications, 1992.

Ross, Jerilyn. *Triumph Over Fear.* Bantam Books, 1994.

Chapter 4: Arthritis

Arthritis Foundation, P.O. Box 19000, Atlanta, GA 30326; (800) 283-7800 — or contact any local affiliate.

Brewer, Earl J., Jr., with Kathy Cochran Angel. *The Arthritis Sourcebook.* Lowell House, 1993.

*Davidson, Paul. *Are You Sure It's Arthritis?* MacMillan, 1985.

Lorig, Kate, with Halsted Holman, David Sobel, Diana Laurent, Virginia Gonzalez, and Marian Minor. *Living A Healthy Life With Chronic Conditions.* Bull Publishing, 1994.

National Arthritis and Musculoskeletal and Skin Diseases Information Clearinghouse, 1 AMS Circle, Bethseda, MD 20892; (301) 495-4484.

Pisetsky, David, with Susan Flamholtz. *The Duke University Medical Center Book of Arthritis.* Fawcett Book Group, 1992.

Sobel, Dava, with Arthur C. Klein. *Arthritis: What Works*. St. Martin's Press, 1992.

Chapter 5: Asthma and Breathing Disorders

American Academy of Allergy, Asthma, and Immunology, 611 East Wells Street, Milwaukee, WI 53202; (800) 822-2762.

American Lung Association, 1740 Broadway, New York, NY 10019-4374; (212) 315-8700 (also many local affiliates).

Asthma and Allergy Foundation of America, 1125 15th St NW #502, Washington, DC 20005; (202) 466-7643/(800) 7-ASTHMA.

Lorig, Kate, with Halsted Holman, David Sobel, Diana Laurent, Virginia Gonzalez, and Marian Minor. *Living A Healthy Life With Chronic Conditions*. Bull Publishing, 1994.

Ostrow, William and Vivian. *All About Asthma*. A. Whitman, 1989.

Chapter 6: Back and Neck

Bean, Constance A. *The Better Back Book*. William Morrow & Co., 1989.

Hochschuler, Stephen. *Back In Shape*. H & M Publishers, 1991.

*Keim, Hugo A. *How To Care For Your Back*. Prentice Hall, 1981.

McIlwain, Harris H., Debra Fulghum Bruce, Joel C. Silverfield, Michael C. Burnette, and Bernard F. Germain. *Winning with Chronic Pain: A Compete Program for Health and Well-being*. Prometheus, 1994.

Sarno, John E. *Healing Back Pain: The Mind Body Connection*. Warner, 1991.

Saunders, H. Duane. *Self-Help Manual for Your Neck*. Available from: Educational Opportunities, 7750 West 78th St., Minneapolis, MN 55439. (612) 944-1656/(800) 654-8357.

Chapter 7: Chronic Fatigue Syndrome

CFIDS Association of America, Inc., P.O. Box 220398, Charlotte, NC 28222-0398; (800) 442-3437. Information Line: (900) 988-2343.

CFS Activation Network: (212) 627-5831

Collinge, William. *Recovering From Chronic Fatigue Syndrome*. Berkley Publishing Group, 1993.

Feiden, Karyn. *Hope and Help for Chronic Fatigue Syndrome*. S&S Publications, 1990.

National Chronic Fatigue Syndrome Association (NCSF), a patient advocacy group, 3521 Broadway #222, Kansas City, MO 64111; (816) 931-4777.

Ostrom, Neeyah. *50 Things You Should Know About The Chronic Fatigue Syndrome Epidemic*. That New Magazine, 1992.

Chapter 8: Depression

DePaulo, J. Raymond, Jr., and Keith R. Ablow. *How to Cope With Depression*. Fawcett, 1990.

Depression and Related Affective Disorders Association, 600 N. Wolfe St., Baltimore, MD 21287-7381; (410) 955-4647.

Jamison, Kay Redfield. *Touched With Fire*. Free Press, 1993.

McGrath, Ellen. *When Feeling Bad is Good*. Bantam, 1994.

Chapter 9: Diabetes

American Diabetes Association, P.O. Box 25757, 1660 Duke St., Alexandria, VA 22314; (703) 549-1500/(800) ADA-DISC.

Anderson, James W. *Diabetes: A Practical New Guide To Healthy Living*. Warner Books, 1981.

Do Your Level Best. A public outreach program of the National Institutes of Health. Free patient information kit available: (800) GET-LEVEL.

Sims, Dorothea F. *Diabetes: Reach for Health and Freedom*. American Diabetes Assn., 1984.

Jovanovic-Peterson, Lois, et al. *A Touch of Diabetes*. Chronimed, 1991.

Chapter 10: Headaches

*Fox, Arnold, with Barry Fox. *DLPA To End Chronic Pain and Depression*. Pocket Books, 1985.

*Gould, Heywood. *Headaches and Health*. St. Martin's Press, 1973.

National Headache Foundation, 5252 N. Webster Ave., Chicago, IL 60625; (312) 878-7715/(800) 843-2256.

*Robbins, Lawrence, and Susan S. Lang. *Headache Help: A Complete Guide to Understanding Headaches and the Medicines that Relieve Them*. Houghton Mifflin, 1995.

Saper, Joel R., with Kenneth R. Magee. *Freedom From Headaches*. S&S Publications, 1987.

Stromfield, Jan, with Anita Weil. *Free Yourself From Headaches*. NAL-Dutton, 1989.

Wyckoff, Betsey. *Overcoming Migraine.* Station Hill Printing, 1991, 1994.

Chapter 11: Heart Disease

American Heart Association, 7272 Greenville Ave., Dallas, TX 75231-4596; (214) 373-6300/(800) 242-8721 (also many local affiliates).

American Yoga Association Hypertension Study 1984: A Summary of Findings. Available from the American Yoga Association, 513 South Orange Avenue, Sarasota, FL 34236.

Bennett, William I., Stephen E. Goldfinger, and G. Timothy Johnson. *Your Good Health, How To Stay Well, And What To Do When You're Not, From Harvard Medical School.* H. U. Publications, 1987.

Cohn, Peter F., and Joan K. Cohn. *Fighting the Silent Killer: How Men and Women Can Prevent and Cope With Heart Disease Today.* A. K. Peters, 1993.

Ornish, Dean. *Dean Ornish's Program for Reversing Heart Disease.* Random House, 1990.

Zaret, Barry, with Marvin Moser and Lawrence S. Cohen. *Yale University School of Medicine Heart Book.* William Morrow & Co., 1992.

Chapter 12: Infertility

Infertility Network Exchange, P.O. Box 204, c/o Ilene Stargot, East Meadow, NY 11554; (516) 794-9772.

Irwin Johnston, Patricia. *Taking Charge of Infertility.* Perspect Indiana, 1994.

Salzer, Linda P. *Surviving Infertility.* Harper Collins, 1991.

Toth, A. *The Fertility Solution.* Grove Atlantic, 1991.

Chapter 13: Insomnia

American Sleep Disorders Association, 1610 14th Street NW #300, Rochester, MN 55901.

Coleman, Richard. *Wide Awake At Three AM By Choice Or By Chance.* Stanford Alumni Assn., 1986.

*Courtenay, Anthea. *Natural Sleep: Beating Insomnia Without Drugs.* Thorsons, 1991.

Hauri, Peter, with Shirley Linde. *No More Sleepless Nights.* John Wiley & Sons, 1990.

Lambly, Peter. *Insomnia and Other Sleeping Problems.* Pinnacle Books, 1989.

*Lamburg, Lynne. *The American Medical Association Guide To Better Sleep.* Random House, 1984.

Sweeney, Donald R. *Overcoming Insomnia.* Bantam Books, 1989.

Chapter 14: Pain Management

American Chronic Pain Association, P.O. Box 850, Rocklin, CA 95677; (916) 632-0922.

*Fox, Arnold. *DLPA To End Chronic Pain and Depression.* Pocket Books, 1985.

McIlwain, Harris M., Debra Fulghum Bruce, Joel C. Silverfield, Michael C. Burnette, and Bernard F. Germain. *Winning WIth Chronic Pain.* Prometheus, 1994.

Chapter 15: PMS and Menopause

Bender, Stephanie D., and Kathleen Kelleher. *PMS: A Positive Program to Gain Control.* Berkley, 1986.

Bender, Stephanie D. *PMS: Questions and Answers.* Berkley, 1989.

Budoff, Penny W. *No More Hot Flashes and Other Good News.* Warner, 1989.

Cutler, Winnifred B., and Delso-Ramon Garcia. *Menopause: A Medical Guide for Women.* Norton, 1993.

Greenwood, Sadja. *Menopause, Naturally: Preparing for the Second Half of Life.* Volcano Press, 1992.

Lark, Susan M. *PMS Self-Help Book.* Celestial Arts, 1989.

Lark, Susan M. *The Menopause Self-Help Book.* Celestial Arts, 1990.

Notelovitz, Morris, with Diana Tonnessen. *Menopause and Midlife Health.* St. Martin's Press, 1994.

Utian, Wulf, and Ruth S. Jacobowitz. *Managing Your Menopause.* Simon & Schuster, 1991.

Chapter 16: Weight Management

Bennett, William I., Stephen E. Goldfinger, and G. Timothy Johnson. *Your Good Health.* Harvard University Press, 1990.

Miller, Peter M. *The Hilton Head Over-35 Diet.* Warner, 1990.

Ornish, Dean. *Eat More, Weigh Less.* Harper/Collins, 1993.

Further information on Yoga is available from the American Yoga Association. If you would like to write to us or obtain a free catalog, call or write:

American Yoga Association
513 South Orange Avenue
Sarasota, FL 34236
Telephone (941) 953-5859
(800) 226-5859
Fax: (941) 953-5859
E-mail: AmYogaAssn@aol.com

We also offer classes in the Cleveland, Ohio, and Sarasota, Florida, areas.

• Books •

The American Yoga Association Beginner's Manual. Complete instructions for over 90 Yoga exercises and breathing techniques; three 10-week curriculum outlines, and chapters on philosophy, stress management, and more.

20-Minute Yoga Workouts: The Perfect Program for the Busy Person. Brief routines that anyone can fit into the busiest schedule. Includes chapters on women's issues, toning and shaping, the "20-minute challenge," and workouts to do when you're away from home.

Easy Does It Yoga For Older People. For those with physical limitations, this book includes instruction in specially adapted Yoga exercises which can be done in a chair or in bed, breathing techniques, and meditation.

The Easy Does It Yoga Trainer's Guide. A complete manual for how to begin teaching the Easy Does It Yoga program to adults with physical limitations due to age, convalescence, substance abuse, injury, or obesity. Intended for health professionals, activities directors, physical therapists, home health aides, and others who work with the elderly or in rehabilitative services.

Meditation. A collection of excerpts from lectures and classes on the subject of meditation, including a section of questions and answers from students.

Reflections of Love. A collection of excerpts from Alice Christensen's lectures and classes on the subject of love.

The Light of Yoga. A chronicle of the unusual circumstances that catapulted Alice Christensen into Yoga practice in the early 1950s, including the teachers and experiences that shaped her first years of study.

The Joy of Celibacy. This booklet examines how the unconscious is influenced by the sexual sell of modern advertising and suggests a five-minute celibacy break to help build awareness and self-knowledge.

Conversations with Swami Lakshmanjoo, Volume I: Aspects of Kashmir Shaivism. Edited transcripts of Alice Christensen's interviews with Swami Lakshmanjoo, talking about his childhood and early years in Yoga, plus some basic concepts in the philosophy of Kashmir Shaivism.

Conversations with Swami Lakshmanjoo, Volume II: The Yamas and Niyamas of Patanjali. Edited transcripts of Alice Christensen's dialogues with Swami Lakshmanjoo about these essential ethical guidelines in Yoga.

• Audiotapes •

Complete Relaxation and Meditation with Alice Christensen. A two-tape audiocassette program that features three guided meditation sessions of varying lengths, including instruction in a seated posture, plus a discussion of meditation experiences.

The "I Love You" Meditation Technique. This technique begins with the experience of a more conscious connection with the breath through love. It then extends this feeling throughout the body and mind in relaxation and meditation. This tape teaches you the beauty of loving yourself and it removes unseen fear.

• Videotapes •

Basic Yoga. A complete introduction to Yoga that includes exercise, breathing, and relaxation and meditation techniques. Provides detailed instruction in all the techniques including variations for more or less flexibility. Features a 30-minute practice session in a Yoga class setting for a convenient routine to do daily.

Conversations with Swami Lakshmanjoo. A set of three videotapes in which Alice Christensen introduces Swami Lakshmanjoo and talks with him about his background, the philosophy of Kashmir Shaivism, and other topics in Yoga. (Some material corresponds to Volume I of the book *Aspects of Kashmir Shaivism* described above.)

The "I Love You" Meditation Technique. (See description under audiotapes).

The Yamas and Niyamas: A Videotape Study Program. A complete set of 24 videotapes of Alice Christensen's comprehensive lectures on the ethical guidelines that form the cornerstone of Yoga philosophy and practice. Includes a study guide.

• About the American Yoga Association •

The American Yoga Association teaches a comprehensive and balanced program of Yoga that includes the Hatha Yoga exercises and breathing techniques as well as meditation. Rather than stressing physical culture for its own sake, our core curriculum acknowledges the deeper possibilities of Yoga by teaching meditation and by encouraging the inner-directed awareness that eventually leads to greater self-knowledge. This reliance on individual experience and feeling is a central theme in the science of Yoga, and it underlies the philosophical system of Kashmir Shaivism which supports our line of teaching.

Our goal is to offer the highest quality yoga instruction possible. There are two American Yoga Association Centers in the United States.

• About the Author •

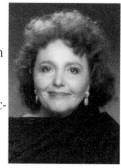

Alice Christensen stands out as a Yoga teacher with the rare ability to make the often-complex ideas and techniques of Yoga accessible to our Western outlook and lifestyle. She established the American Yoga Association in 1968, then the first and only nonprofit organization in the United States dedicated to education in Yoga.

Alice has consistently presented Yoga in a clear, classical manner for over 40 years. She presents Yoga without dogma or prescription, as a potent avenue for individual inquiry. She has designed programs of Yoga that can be used to enhance any lifestyle. Whether the goal is to maintain health or to explore the nature of the self, her programs can be used to achieve a wide range of goals.